IMPORTANT NOTICE

Do not use this book until you have read these pages.

You have in your hands one half of the system that will change your life. To achieve success it is essential that you download the other half of this system from the Hay House website:

hayhouse.com/mckenna

and use the audio and video sessions that complete it.

This is not just a book to read, it is part of a life-changing solution. This book is the first essential element of the system. The audio and video sessions are just as important: you must use both the book and the audio and video sessions to achieve permanent success.

The sessions contain everything I would do if I were working with you personally. They include simple, powerful psychological techniques and a hypnotic trance that strengthen the power of your subconscious mind to guide your success.

The sessions are really easy to download onto your computer or smartphone, just a few clicks, then a few minutes later, you will have me there whenever you need, to help you make the changes you want.

Intellectual knowledge is not the same as real change, so you cannot expect lasting results if you only read this book. You must download and use the psychological techniques and guided hypnosis to achieve permanent, positive change.

In hypnotic trance your unconscious is highly receptive to positive intentions. It is not the same as sleep; it is a wonderful state of deep relaxation, like a daydream or meditation, and even though you are deeply relaxed, if for any reason you need to awaken, you will do so with all the resources you need.

The audio and video techniques are not just essential, they are also enjoyable and rewarding. In fact, many people use them over and over to reinforce their new mind-set and enhance their success.

Ensure your success now. Go online now to:

hayhouse.com/mckenna

1. Input the product ID and download code shown below (also found on the card at the front of this book) and then download the free sessions right now:

    Product ID: 3116

    Download code: mckenna

2. Use the audio hypnosis session every night just before you go to sleep, for the next seven days.

3. Use the video sessions to ensure lasting success!

I CAN MAKE YOU SLEEP

PAUL MCKENNA, PH.D.

EDITED BY HUGH WILLBOURN, PH.D.

HAY HOUSE, INC.
Carlsbad, California • New York City
London • Sydney • Johannesburg
Vancouver • Hong Kong • New Delhi

Published and distributed in the United States by: Hay House, Inc.:
www.hayhouse.com® • **Published and distributed in Australia by:**
Hay House Australia Pty. Ltd.: www.hayhouse.com.au • **Published and
distributed in the United Kingdom by:** Hay House UK, Ltd.: www.
hayhouse.co.uk • **Published and distributed in the Republic of South
Africa by:** Hay House SA (Pty), Ltd.: www.hayhouse.co.za • **Distributed
in Canada by:** Raincoast Books: www.raincoast.com • **Published in
India by:** Hay House Publishers India: www.hayhouse.co.in

Cover design: Alex Tuppen

Previously published in Great Britain by Bantam Press, a division of
Transworld Publishers, ISBN: 9780593055380.

Cataloging-in-Publication Data is on file at the Library of Congress

Tradepaper ISBN: 978-1-4019-4899-3

10 9 8 7 6 5 4 3 2 1
1st Hay House edition, June 2016

Printed in the United States of America

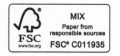

I CAN MAKE
YOU SLEEP

WARNING

IMPORTANT: ABOUT THE HYPNOTIC TRANCE DOWNLOAD

Accompanying this book is a hypnotic trance download that will help you to reestablish your natural cycle of deep, restful sleep at night and refreshed alertness during the day. Use the hypnotic trance when you go to bed at night. Use it as many nights as you wish to help you sleep and to program your mind to sleep better and deeper in the future. You can find the details on the special card at the front of the book.

Your mind is like a computer. It has its own software that organizes all the automatic processes of your mind and your body. I have worked with many people with insomnia over many years, and I have learned that almost all their problems have arisen because their natural sleep cycle has been disrupted. The hypnotic trance is designed to restore your natural cycle of sleep and alertness.

As you listen to the hypnotic trance regularly at night, you will reinforce all the improvements you are making by reading this book and practicing the exercises in it.

Use the hypnotic trance as often as you wish to enhance your ability to sleep, but remember only to use it in bed when you are ready to sleep.

• • •

•

CHAPTER 1

Welcome to the World of Regular, Deep, Refreshing Sleep

Welcome to the World of Regular, Deep, Refreshing Sleep

The system in this book and in the hypnotic trance and video sessions will make a huge improvement to your life. If you've suffered from insomnia or from disruption to your sleep, then I have written this book for you! This system will do more than help you sleep longer, it will also significantly improve the quality of your sleep. Human beings spend approximately 30 percent of their life asleep, so almost a third of your entire existence is about to become significantly better.

Every human being has a natural inbuilt ability to sleep deeply and for long periods of time. We are going to reestablish your sleep cycle so that you truly enjoy that natural ability.

Recent research has shown that we do not all need eight hours of sleep every night; some people only need five or six hours. However much you sleep, what matters is that you are truly rested and refreshed. As you use this book, together we will improve the quantity and the quality of your sleep. Whether your sleep gets longer or deeper or both, it will become more refreshing and satisfying, so overall a third of your life is about to get better!

I know the frustration of not getting a good night's sleep and I know that I can help you. There are different ways that people experience sleeping problems or insomnia—some find it difficult to get to sleep, other people wake up frequently during the night, others wake too early in the morning. Some people have a mixture of all those difficulties, and some people never enjoy feeling truly rested, however much they sleep.

For you this is all going to change, right now. Whatever your problem was with sleeping, from now on, your sleep will start to improve. One of the best things about this system is that you don't have to "believe" in it, you don't have to have willpower. You simply have to follow my instructions.

Everything You Need Is Here

The system you are about to use has taken over 20 years to develop. Everything that is in this book, hypnotic trance, and video downloads is exactly what I would do with you if we were sitting together doing a personal session. In fact, during the reading of this book you may find yourself feeling sleepy.

There are two reasons for this. First, simply by reading about how your sleep can get better and deeper we are focusing your mind on sleep and activating all your unconscious associations to successfully falling asleep. Many people find that reading this book makes them feel a bit sleepy or that their attitudes to sleep begin to transform, because it has been written in a special hypnotic language. The formula of the writing makes the brain begin to process ideas to reconnect to your basic ability to sleep. As you make sense of what I am saying your mind creates a specific sequence of ideas that puts positive suggestions into your unconscious mind.

I've worked with many people over the years helping them to change habits, and the research into my techniques shows that they work for most people most of the time. However, I am always interested in why my approach doesn't work for some people, and interestingly it's always the same reason:

They didn't follow the instructions.

This can be for any number of reasons. Maybe they were distracted, or they tried the techniques just once or twice and forgot to repeat them.

The point is if they don't follow the instructions, they are not using the system. It is important to explain straight away that the system in this book and hypnotic trance works by installing the habits of success in your mind. One of the methods by which we do this is repetition, so if you want to improve the length and quality of your sleep, you must follow all my instructions—including the repetitions. If you don't follow them, you are not using the system.

Many people find that their sleep improves radically within a few days. Even though this may happen to you, keep using all the techniques. Establishing regular, refreshing sleep is the result of changing many small processes that all add up to work together. Keep following all the rules until they become second nature and use the exercises as often as you wish, and after a few weeks you will find out which is your favorite way to go to sleep.

Sleep is a simple experience created by a multitude of complex factors. For a few people it is just one of the changes I suggest, or just one of the exercises, that makes a huge difference. And of course, most of the time we can't tell exactly which were the changes that were critical for your sleep improvement. That is why it is necessary to follow the whole system. After all, it doesn't matter if you do not know which change it was you made that makes you sleep better. All that matters is that you sleep deeper and longer and better and feel more refreshed, more relaxed, and more alert during the day. Some people find it helpful to reread this book many times as well in order to reinforce the learning.

We are going to start this book by changing simple habits and improving your sleep environment. Then later in the book I will show you some powerful psychological techniques that you can use to go to sleep and stay asleep longer and deeper.

Relax, You Can Do It

If you have been unable to sleep, it is not your fault. It's the fault of your programming. You mind is like a computer, and when you learn to do something you store it as a program in your unconscious mind. That is what a habit is. So being unable to sleep at night is simply the product of some bad habits.

When a baby is born it alternates between sleeping and waking on a very short cycle of a few hours. One of the first things it does is build up longer periods of sleep and longer periods of wakefulness. Babies do this quite naturally by means of a built-in mechanism that reacts to the light during the day and the darkness at night. Babies still need to sleep a fair amount during the day because they are growing and learning so fast, but as we get older we sleep more and more at night and less and less during the day.

Learning to regulate our sleep is one of the first things we do, so we can do it again simply by letting that natural tendency take over again. That's what we are going to do over the next few weeks. Very soon you will have developed the habit of sleeping well.

As you start using the techniques in this book it's important to remember to focus your mind on what is working. I had a client once who was suffering from insomnia. Some weeks after our first session I asked him, "How is it going?" He replied, "I am afraid I'm not cured." So I asked him, "But how much better is your sleep?" And he said, "Oh, about 80 percent." Some people tend to search for what isn't working, rather than what is. Often because they are natural problem-solvers, so they have to search for what's wrong. This is a useful skill, and I have a technique later to make sure that skill can be preserved and you can also get to sleep. As you use these exercises it is important to notice how things improve so that your mind is focused on your successes.

You might find your natural sleep pattern does not have the timing you expect. Over the next few weeks I want you to focus on what is getting better even if it is happening in an unexpected way. How much longer are you sleeping? Or is it the quality of your sleep that is improving? As you follow my instructions, do you find yourself going to bed earlier or later than you expected?

What Makes This System Work?

As you read this book I will take you through each of the different areas of your life which affect your sleep and show you how to set them all up so that you sleep better and better.

If you forget one of the exercises or have a bad night, don't worry—nobody does it perfectly at first. Getting it wrong is part of the learning process; just start again and carry on. Because there are many different factors affecting your sleep, the improvement is very rarely a gradual, straightforward increase in length and depth of sleep. Some people find their sleep improves within a few nights, but for many there are periods of no change followed by sudden improvements, then one or two less good nights, then patches of smooth improvements or more sudden gains. This happens because lots of different subsystems of your body and mind are changing at the same time.

From a practical point of view these details don't matter. Just keep following the system even if you have two whole weeks of great, deep sleep and then one slightly shorter night. Keep following the rules and the average time of sleep and the quality of your sleep will get better and better until you naturally sleep deeply and continuously each night.

How to Program Your Mind

This system is unique because it is designed to use both your conscious and your unconscious mind to restore the fundamental sleep cycle. By using both parts of your mind you are doubling the efficiency of the system. Let me explain a little bit about the two parts of your mind.

Your Conscious Mind

This is the mind that you actively and deliberately think with all day long. It is the internal voice that you think of as "me." But while the conscious mind certainly has its uses, it is extremely limited in what it can accomplish on its own. Studies have shown that it can only hold a handful of ideas at any one time. That's why throughout your life your conscious mind is assisted by the power and capacity of your other, larger mind—the unconscious mind.

Your Unconscious Mind

Your unconscious mind is the larger mind; it is the part of you that ultimately controls every aspect of your behavior. It keeps your heart beating, your brain thinking, and your body healthy and energized. It stores and runs all the "programs" of automatic behavior that you use to live your life.

The unconscious mind is like having an "autopilot" function in the brain that allows us to do multiple things simultaneously without having to concentrate on all of them at once. For example, when you were a child you had to concentrate consciously in order to learn to tie your shoelaces properly, using your conscious mind. But now that your unconscious mind has learned the sequence of moves, it can direct your hands and you do not need to pay attention to the process consciously anymore.

These programs ("habits") are useful because they free our conscious minds to think about other things. Learning to drive a car involves learning lots of little processes like scanning the road, signaling, accelerating, braking, turning, and so forth. As you practice each one, and turn the sequence of perceptions and moves into automatic programs, your unconscious mind takes over the specific actions involved in driving, and you monitor the process without having to think about how you accelerate, turn, signal, and so on. You can just get in the car and decide where you want to go. If something unusual or dangerous happens, you can react instantly because you don't have to think about how to brake or steer or accelerate. You can do it without thinking.

It is great learning to drive, but some of the habits we have learned are less useful. Because the unconscious mind simply learns things that are repeated, whether or not we really want to learn them, it is possible to learn and install a bad habit completely by accident. In fact, insomnia is just that: a habit.

No one gets it deliberately. It doesn't mean you are mad, bad, or broken. People only learn the habit of insomnia by accident. Unfortunately, many people do not realize it is a habit that can be changed, and they don't know that actually it is quite straightforward, and that's what we are going to discover as you use this system over the next few weeks.

Using Both Parts of Your Mind

There are some functions of the unconscious mind that are preprogrammed, such as breathing. We don't need to learn how to do it—as soon as we are born we start to breathe. Nevertheless, we can choose to speed up our breathing or slow it down. We can't stop it entirely though. If you try to hold your breath forever, you will fail, because the basic instincts in the unconscious will take over and literally force you to breathe.

Some of the other basic functions cannot be directly controlled at all. For example, while you can choose to speed up your breathing, you cannot simply choose to speed up your heartbeat. However, we can influence our heartbeat through the power of imagination. If we imagine walking down a dark alley late at night and hearing footsteps behind us, our hearts will almost certainly speed up. In the same way, if you vividly imagine a scene that you find calm and relaxing, such as lying on a warm beach hearing the distant rhythmic crash and hiss of the waves, or dozing on a comfortable sofa in front of a log fire and watching the flames flicker, or walking through a quiet and beautiful forest with the light dappled through the trees, your heartbeat will become calm and steady and your body chemistry will release endorphins and other hormones that make you feel calm and relaxed.

In other words, changing how you think and what you think can cause the state of your body to change. Some of the powerful techniques in this book involve

the use of imagination techniques to reprogram the unconscious mind. With carefully selected imagery and
networks of association we can stimulate changes in the
neurological and hormonal patterns that facilitate sleep.

To benefit from the system all you have to do is
follow the instructions. Read the book—at least twice,
preferably three times, and do each of the exercises.
Make sure you do them all—even the ones that seem
at first as if you may not like them as much as others.
Some people benefit most from the exercises they find a
little difficult at first. That is not so surprising; really—
the better you are at something, the less you need to
practice it—and conversely if you find something very
difficult, it indicates that there is a lot there for you to
learn so that it becomes more easy.

How to Use the Hypnotic Trance Download

This book comes with a hypnotic trance that will help you go to sleep, and with repeated use it will help you restore your natural, healthy sleep patterns.

The trance is specially recorded so that the hypnotic suggestions are taken up by the unconscious mind, and the structure and timing of the hypnotic trance are carefully calibrated to enhance your sleep cycle. But I have discovered that, on top of that, just using hypnosis leads to improved sleep. When I teach hypnosis seminars my students go in and out of trance several times a day for a week. I noticed that many of them report at the end of the week that they are sleeping better and deeper than they have for years.

I've been helping people to sleep better for many years, and some of them have found that just using the trance has been all they need to improve their sleep patterns permanently.

I want to be 100 percent certain that your sleep will improve, so I want you to use the hypnotic trance and I want you to follow every instruction and use every exercise in this book. That means that whatever your problem was, you will improve your sleep. Also, you will be able to sleep well even if there are nights when you can't listen to the hypnotic trance.

I believe one of the reasons that people have such a high success rate with my change work is simply that we cover every angle. I've looked at all the reasons people had sleep problems, and when you use the whole of this system there is something that helps everyone.

The ideal time to listen to the hypnotic trance is in bed as you go to sleep.

As you use it regularly, you will reinforce all the changes you are making and boost your natural sleep cycle. When you listen to the hypnotic trance you don't have to make any effort at all. You don't have to believe in anything, you just need to hear the words and sounds on the hypnotic trance and let your mind take what it needs. You can listen but you don't need to try to remember anything or even try to understand it. All that is necessary is simply to hear it so that the unconscious mind extracts from it all it needs to help you sleep better and better.

Hypnotic trance is not the same as sleep. You will hear all the words on the hypnotic trance and your awareness may change, but you will be able to rouse yourself if necessary. However, you will also find it much, much easier to slip into sleep from trance. You can also use the hypnotic trance if you wake up during the night.

Whether you drift off very rapidly into sleep or whether you listen to the hypnotic trance all the way through doesn't matter. There is a wide variety of natural states of relaxation you can experience in addition to sleep, and while you do that I will reprogram your unconscious mind to sleep regularly and deeply just like reinstalling a program on a computer. Your mind is like a computer in many ways. It has its own software that helps you to organize your thinking and behavior. Having worked with all sorts of people with different problems over many years, I have learned that almost all problems stem from the same cause—programs have been installed in the unconscious mind that have undesirable outcomes. Sometimes the program was installed accidentally like a computer virus, other times people are still running programs to solve problems that no longer exist. Either way, the solution is the same. Remove the old program and reinstall a new, clean, better version.

What Can I Expect?

As you use this system over the next few weeks your sleep cycle will be greatly improved. After that, depending on many factors, not least your starting point, there may be room for some more improvement, or it may be that you simply need to spend more time following all the rules carefully so that you embed all the new learnings in the unconscious mind to keep the unconscious mind delivering better sleep.

After two months you will find that your sleep cycle has become fairly robust. That means that even if for some reason you have to stay up later or your sleep is interrupted, your sleep cycle should reestablish itself easily within a couple of nights. If for any reason at all your sleep becomes disrupted again, go back to following all the instructions, using all the exercises, and listening to the hypnotic trance for at least a week. This will ensure that the momentum of improvement is restored.

As we will see in the next chapter, sleep is a function of a number of ongoing cycles, some of which run over many days. Therefore, we cannot change your long-term sleeping patterns in a single night. Although you can have very rapid improvement very swiftly, we have to work over a longer period in order to reset the ongoing rhythm of your sleep cycle.

Our brains and bodies are running thousands of different interlocking cycles to keep us alive and healthy. These processes replenish the energy in our muscles, they build and repair the cells in our bodies, and they organize our memory and understanding. The sleep function is involved in all of these. We have to help your mind and body to adjust the power and timing of these interlocking cycles so that the major pattern of sleep becomes more unified, more powerful, and more robust.

I will explain this in more detail and show you exactly how you can enhance that cycle in the next chapter. The point I need to make here is that the process has to be done over a sequence of nights. We can't just stop the processes in your body, adjust them, and then start them up again—we have to adjust them all while they are in motion.

There are three main ways we do this:

- *We eliminate sleep disruptors.*

- *We introduce sleep enhancers.*

- *We optimize your environment to maintain the improvements.*

In the following chapters we will explore each of the areas that can affect your sleep and deal with them all one by one. In each area I will show you how to eliminate all the disrupting factors, how to insert sleep enhancers, and how to optimize the environment to foster and maintain improvement in the long term. Follow the whole system, do all the exercises, and your sleep will get a whole lot better.

It doesn't matter how many problems you have had with your sleep; if you follow every single step of this system, your sleep will improve. The improvement may be sudden or it may be gradual. But even if you experience the positive effects very rapidly, it is important to keep following the rules and to try out all the exercises. We are in the business of improving your sleep for life, not just for a few nights, and therefore we need to deal with all the possible causes of disruption so that the natural cycle of sleep runs smoothly week after week.

Read the whole of the book as many times as you need to and do ALL the exercises.

To truly improve your sleep it is better to make a little extra effort than to miss correcting the one thing that will allow you to create a great pattern of long, deep, restful sleep you can rely on for the rest of your life.

Medical Matters

A number of medical conditions can interfere with sleeping patterns.

If you have any symptoms that lead you to think you might have a medical condition, you should consult your doctor. However, that does not mean you cannot improve your sleep.

In many cases, sleeping better can be a major help in the healing process. For example, poor sleep can be a symptom of depression. Sleeping better is one of the two most effective remedies for depression; the other is exercise.

In other cases, such as arthritis, people are kept awake by chronic pain. Again, this system will help you sleep better even if you suffer from chronic pain, but you should not change your treatment regime for any medical condition without consulting your doctor.

The following medical conditions have been associated with poor sleep. Even when your sleep improves radically you should still consult your doctor as you would normally for appropriate help with any of these conditions: depression, restless leg syndrome, chronic pain, Parkinson's disease, heart disease, hypertension, hyperthyroidism, asthma, allergies, and attention deficit disorder.

What If I Already Use Sleep Medication?

You should always consult your doctor if you have any concerns about your medication or if you wish to change or reduce your use of prescription drugs. Many doctors believe that in an ideal world medication to help people sleep should not be used for more than two weeks at a time, but for different reasons there are a lot of people who use such medication routinely. Unfortunately, this can cause habituation to the drugs, and people can become reliant on medication. Worse still, the effectiveness of the drugs reduces with continuous use.

I have used sleep medication for jet lag and found it effective. But I know that after a few nights of use it begins to be less effective. That is why I am so much in favor of the system in this book.

If you wish to stop using medication for sleep, you should do so only under medical supervision. Use this book and hypnotic trance as well and they will help you to set up a robust, natural pattern of regular, refreshing sleep.

• • •

CHAPTER 2

•

The First Key to
Sleep: Timing

The First Key to Sleep: Timing

You are an amazing human being. On the one hand the complexity of the systems and processes that keep us alive is astonishing; on the other hand there is a wonderful simplicity about the way we can use the systems at our disposal to live healthily and sleep well.

There has been an enormous amount of research into sleep over the last 50 years. I'm just going to tell you some of the key findings so you can understand how your sleep will improve and how the rules and exercises work.

Sleep and the Body

Our bodies and brains are continually working. Whether you are asleep or awake, your lungs keep breathing and your heart keeps beating. Hundreds of other complex processes are also in continual motion to maintain, refuel, and repair the millions of different cells that make up our bodies. Digestion converts food to energy, and the organs of the body work night and day to keep us healthy and fit. But all these processes do not run at the same speed all the time. Just as we breathe slower and deeper when we sleep and faster when we exercise, each process adjusts and evolves over time. In fact, many of the major processes, such as cell repair and growth, work in cycles. These consist of series of events that repeat themselves over and over again. The maintenance of the whole body is run by means of a cycle of repeating processes.

However, there's a little more to it, because these different cycles are all connected and constantly adjusting in relation to each other—and on top of that, everything we choose to do affects these cycles.

Here's an example: if you go for a run, a hormone called adrenaline is released. This helps to speed up your heart and direct blood to your major muscles so they can extract extra oxygen, which releases energy to power you along. At the same time your breathing gets deeper and more vigorous to push more oxygen into your blood. Running soon makes you hot, so you start to sweat to prevent overheating.

When you stop running, your body releases endorphins that make you feel good and help you to relax. Then over the next few hours yet more hormones are released to trigger the repair and refueling of your muscles.

Running is a natural activity for which evolution has prepared us, so the body is well prepared to go through the sequence of activating these cycles. During the day, we trigger cycles one after another—eating, working, walking, thinking, talking, and so forth. By the end of the day we have used many different capacities of our mind and body and the whole system needs some time to repair and refuel and to integrate the learning of the day. And that is what sleep does for us.

The Natural Sleep Mechanism Within You

Sleep is so important for our health that our bodies force us to sleep at least the minimum amount necessary to keep us going. But if your sleep is poor, you may have had little more than that, so you could have been getting stressed, tired, or run down.

The reason some people fail to improve their sleep is that they home in on one cause and try to fix that—but there are different possible causes, and for most people their sleep disruption has more than one.

And just as there are many causes of disruption, to develop a robust pattern of sleeping well night after night we have to realign many different patterns and cycles in the body. Even though that seems like a big task, there is a very straightforward way to do it.

One of the reasons the approach I am outlining in this book works so well is because it treats the whole system. If someone fixes only one part, they could have a good night's sleep and then be woken because another problem is still there and hasn't been fixed. In this book, we restore the basic rhythm. As you read this book and do the exercises you will clear out all the disrupting factors and install sleep enhancers for your own natural cycle of sleep and wakefulness so that it runs cleanly and properly.

How Your Sleep Cycle Works

A cycle is simply a pattern that repeats over and over again with a particular rhythm. The daily cycle of sleep and wakefulness is one of the biggest natural cycles in your life.

You could think of it like a swing. Imagine a home-made swing, a little plank suspended on two ropes from the branch of a tree. Imagine pushing a child on that swing. With each push you give them you add to their momentum, and each push carries them higher. The higher they go, the faster the swing goes as they come down again, and the momentum carries them further up the other side. But if you stop pushing them, they will gradually lose momentum and, little by little, the swing will get lower and lower and eventually will come to a halt.

Pushing a child on a swing is a gentle process. All we need to do is give the child a little push at the right time, just as they are beginning to swing down again. But think of what happens if you get your timing wrong. If you leave it too late, the child is accelerating away from you and you almost have to run after them to push at all—and you have hardly any effect. Or if you try to start pushing too soon, you feel the weight of the child against you and the child comes to a sudden halt. Even the simplest swing can get out of time, and it can look quite complicated if your attempt to correct adds another twist or spin.

That is all that has happened when your sleep cycle is disrupted—the rhythm of the swing has got out of synch. There is nothing profoundly wrong or bad or broken. You are not essentially different from other human beings.

Your sleep cycle is like that swing—once upon a time you had a nice simple back-and-forth swing—up and down, up and down—sleep deep at night and nice and bright during the day. Then you suffered from having that rhythm disrupted. So our job is to get a regular rhythm going again.

What Actually Happens When You Sleep

Scientists have used EEG (electroencephalogram) machines to monitor the brainwave activity of people sleeping and discovered that we all go through several different phases of sleep several times a night. The phases of sleep have been labeled several different ways over the years, but nowadays in sleep laboratories researchers recognize essentially three distinct types.

Light Sleep

When you fall asleep the first phase of sleep you enter is called "light sleep." The characteristic brain waves of this phase are quite fast. If you whisper someone's name while they are in light sleep, a response appears on the EEG: a pattern that sleep researchers call a k-complex. It is the tall spike in the wave pattern below.

Slow Wave Sleep

The second type of sleep is called "slow wave" sleep, because brain waves become slower and more regular. Usually we go into this phase of sleep about 20 minutes after we fall asleep and stay there for about two hours. In this phase our bodies are rejuvenated. Since there is no demand to expend energy on the outside, the body takes the opportunity to repair itself and to activate the immune system that fights disease and restores health. Experiments have demonstrated that these two hours of deep, slow wave sleep are essential for our health, and even if the possibility of sleeping is drastically reduced, the unconscious mind makes sure we get these two hours.

REM Sleep

The third type of sleep is known as REM sleep. REM stands for "rapid eye movement." In this phase your eyes can be seen moving beneath your eyelids and your brain activity is very similar to the waking state—but you don't move around, because your body is completely relaxed. Further experiments have demonstrated that the activity of the brain during REM sleep leads to improved performance of learned tasks. It is as though the unconscious mind uses the time to organize, file, and install the new patterns you have learned during the previous day. REM sleep is the lightest type. People often wake up in the morning directly from REM sleep.

If you do that, then typically you will find you remember your dreams quite vividly.

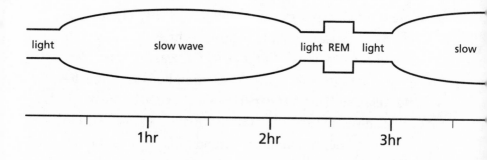

The Whole Sleep Cycle

In a normal sleep pattern we start in light sleep for about 20 minutes, then go into slow wave sleep for about two hours.* Then our brain waves speed up and we spend about 20 minutes in REM sleep. Then our brain waves slow down again and we go through light sleep to slow wave sleep again. We don't spend so long in slow wave sleep the second time. Then once again we go up through light sleep to REM sleep. In an ordinary night we go through this cycle three or four times.

| light | slow wave | light | REM | light | slow |

| 1hr | 2hr | 3hr |

*Earlier researchers divided light sleep into phases 1 and 2, and slow wave sleep into phases 3 and 4. However, more recently, many researchers in sleep laboratories distinguish mainly between light, slow wave, and REM sleep.

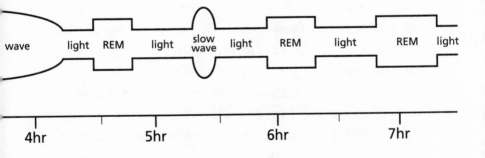

So How Does This Affect Me?

Well, knowing how we move up and down through light, slow wave, and REM sleep cycles helps us to understand why a good number of people sometimes wake up about three hours after they go to sleep. They have had their essential two hours of slow wave sleep, they go up into REM, and then they awaken. They have a perfectly healthy, normal sleep cycle, but the level of the cycle is set too "high," so instead of going back down from REM into light and then deep sleep again, they overshoot and become a little too alert in their REM phase and wake up. There are many different reasons why this can happen. Stress and alcohol can both cause it, for example. Once you remove the initial cause, then all you need to do is to reset the "level" of the cycle. We do that through recalibrating the timing, as you will see below.

Some people who come into sleep laboratories to be examined are convinced that they never sleep a wink, night after night. Every time such people are hooked up to EEG machines that measure brain waves, it turns out that they are getting the essential two hours of deep sleep. However, it may be very fragmented. Many of them take a long time to fall asleep and when they wake up they forget they were ever asleep. Some dream about being awake before they wake up, which is even more misleading.

In fact, it takes extreme conditions and the cooperation of a team of assistants to keep anyone continually awake for more than two and a half days, because the unconscious mind insists on putting you to sleep. If someone tries to go for days without sleep, they fall into what are known as "micro-sleeps": short periods of sleep, a few seconds to a few minutes long. In experiments when people are deliberately kept awake for two days or more they begin to experience irrational fears and mood swings and even hallucinations. Luckily, as soon as they are permitted to get some sleep, all these symptoms disappear. If someone has been awake for too long, when they fall asleep they go directly into slow wave sleep, and after a slightly longer and deeper sleep than usual they are back to normal.

How to Reset Your Sleep Cycle

By now perhaps you are thinking, "All this science is very interesting, but how is it going to help me sleep?" After all, millions of people sleep perfectly well without knowing anything about their brain waves. The point is that sleep is one phase in a set of interconnected cycles that run continuously throughout the day and night. These cycles are going on all the time, so you can't simply stop them and start again. In order to sort out your sleep we need to "nudge" the whole set of cycles in the right direction.

We can do that by changing the bits we can reach easily: what time you wake up, and what you do while you are awake.

The first thing we need to do is to add more energy to the cycle of sleep and wakefulness. We need to add this momentum to the sleep cycle in the right place—a bit like pushing the child on the swing at the right time.

In other words, we want to make the urge to go to sleep more powerful. To do that, we need to give it an extra "push." The first way to do this is to increase your readiness to sleep by bringing forward the end of the sleep cycle. We cannot directly control when you fall asleep, but we can control when you wake up, and when you wake up earlier, it pulls forward the time at which your body is ready to go to bed at the end of the day. This is the first way to add momentum to your sleep cycle and get it back on track. This is like catching the swing at the very top of the swinging and pulling it a bit higher, so that when it swings back down again it has more energy and it goes a little faster and a little farther.

"Push" Number 1

Get up half an hour earlier than your usual wake-up time.

If you normally get up at 7:00 A.M., for the next few weeks get up at 6:30 A.M. This may not sound like much, or it may sound a bit too much if you have been losing a lot of sleep, but clinical research has demonstrated that this is the single most effective strategy for curing insomnia. No matter how much or how little you've slept, get up at your new earlier waking time. One reason this is so important is that if the body gets used to catching up on sleep late in the morning, it does not prepare properly for sleep at the beginning of the night. Your unconscious mind, and your body's rhythms, determine when you go to sleep, but you can consciously choose when you're going to wake up. When you move the waking-up time, the rest of the cycle has to move as well.

Social scientists have demonstrated that it is easier to achieve the change you desire if you make a commitment to yourself by writing down your goals. So please do that now—write down your new getting-up time on a piece of paper or card and put it next to your bed. And while you are there, adjust your alarm clock. Set it half an hour earlier.

Push number one gives extra momentum to the cycle. Now we need to make sure that at the other end of the cycle you do not rush too fast to get to sleep. Continuing our comparison with the swing, you must wait for the swing to reach you, not try to grab at it before it has arrived.

"Push" Number 2

Go to bed only when you are sleepy.
It is as simple as that. If you aren't sleepy, don't go to bed. However tired you might want to be, or think you ought to be, don't go to bed unless you actually feel sleepy. Stay up and read, get on with all the jobs and tasks you've been putting off, and go to bed only when you feel really sleepy. You have already been surviving on not much sleep and you won't get any more by trying to force it. When your body needs it, it will let you know. This means you should never say things like "I'd better go to bed now as I need my sleep" if you don't feel sleepy. Only when you feel sleepy is it correct to decide to go to bed. When you first start using this system you may find that you are up much later than usual. Don't worry, that is perfectly normal. After a few days of going to bed late and getting up half an hour earlier, you will find that your natural sleepiness begins to show up earlier in the evening.

As you use these two "pushes" night after night it builds up the pressure to sleep and gets the natural swing going more and more smoothly.

There is one more "push" to make as well, which is like a child kicking their legs as they swing down to add momentum to the swing. This extra "push" is a matter of keeping the momentum in the swing and not getting distracted. In order to build up the "readiness to sleep" you must stay awake all day every day. If we let ourselves nod off during the day, the natural rhythm we are building up is disrupted.

"Push" Number 3

Don't take naps during the day.
Your appetite for sleep is rather like your appetite for food. If you graze on snacks all day long, you don't have much of an appetite at mealtimes, but if you don't snack between mealtimes, you have a healthy appetite when you sit down to dinner. So do not take a nap or go to bed during the day. Only go to bed at night, and only when you feel sleepy.

Of course, people who already sleep well may not be following all these rules, but you need to improve your sleep so to be sure we restore your natural sleep cycle you do need to follow them all.

In a Nutshell

Sleep is a rhythmic pattern of light and deep sleep. To restore your natural rhythm we give the cycle three "pushes":

PUSH NUMBER 1

GET UP HALF AN HOUR EARLIER THAN YOUR USUAL WAKE-UP TIME.

PUSH NUMBER 2

GO TO BED ONLY WHEN YOU ARE SLEEPY.

PUSH NUMBER 3

DON'T TAKE NAPS DURING THE DAY.

• • •

CHAPTER 3

•

Small Changes That Make a Big Difference to Your Sleep

Small Changes That Make a Big Difference to Your Sleep

There is a strong correlation between being overweight and having poor sleeping patterns, so as you want to sleep, staying at your optimum weight is a good idea. I learned a lot about losing weight from running weight-loss seminars, and I wrote a book about it. In spite of all the different things that are written about it, if you need to lose weight it is a simple process. One part of it is simply increasing the exercise you get. And everyone, whether or not they are losing weight, benefits from simple, regular exercise.

Why? The answer is simple: our bodies are designed to do a certain amount of physical effort every day. Even 50 years ago it was difficult to live without having to get exercise such as walking, doing manual work, housework, or fetching and carrying. However with today's modern, mechanized lifestyle it is quite possible to live without ever fully exerting yourself. This is unhealthy for two simple reasons:

1. The body has muscles that are designed to work every day, and if they don't, the muscles get weaker and our body begins to store energy as fat.

2. Exercise is one of the best ways to flush out the toxins that stress can create in the body.

But even more interesting for us, as well as being a third reason why it is better for your health:

3. It is scientifically proven that exercise improves sleep.

So a simple, gentle increase in the amount of exercise you get can reduce stress, reduce weight, and improve your sleep.

How to Make Exercise Easy

A very obvious benefit of exercise is that it makes you physically tired, and we all know that tiredness helps you sleep better. But there is more to it than that. Sleep researchers have found that while any exercise is good, it is even better if you finish your exercise at least three hours before you go to bed, because the body needs a certain amount of time to metabolize all the hormones that are released while you are exercising.

Also, exercise raises your core body temperature and it takes a few hours for it to fall again. Furthermore, when you go to sleep your body temperature falls even further, and it is at its lowest about 3 A.M. So if your body temperature is naturally falling, it is easy for it to simply carry on falling as you go to bed to sleep.

When I mention exercise, lots of people think I'm talking about joining a gym or pumping iron. Exercise is just using your muscles. In my weight-loss seminars there are always people there who say they never exercise. So I ask them, "How did you get here? Did someone carry you? Don't you get out of bed in the morning? Don't you walk around the house?" All movement is exercise, so you are already exercising, you just might not be doing enough.

Dr. James Hill has done a fascinating study that revealed that the average number of steps taken per day by women between the ages of 18 and 50 was only a little over 5,000. (For men, the average was closer to 6,000 steps a day.) Even more intriguingly, the study revealed that people who were overweight took 1,500 to 2,000 fewer steps a day than those who maintained a healthy weight. That is approximately equivalent to a 15-minute walk.

In other words:

Only 2,000 extra steps a day can make the difference between being overweight and being fit.

If you want to know how many steps you already walk each day, you can buy a simple pedometer (step counter) that attaches to your belt and costs just a few dollars. Rather than join a gym and go at it too hard then give up two weeks later, make it easy to succeed. Build up your steps a little more each day.

What really convinced me of this was a friend of mine who used my weight-loss system years ago and lost 70 pounds. Interestingly, he never went to the gym once. However, he started walking more, rushing about, and getting things done. It's important to remember that no matter how much you want to change, it will still only happen one day at a time. You don't need to start a formal exercise routine, just move your body whenever you get the chance. Take the stairs instead of the elevator. Park farther away from the office and walk 2,000 extra steps to work. Move. Dance. Play sports. Have fun. You only have one body, so you might as well enjoy it!

Sleep Apnea

This is a condition often, but not exclusively, associated with being overweight. It causes very poor quality sleep.

In sleep apnea, the sleeper temporarily stops breathing and then restarts, usually with a loud snore. The stoppage is caused by the airway to the lungs closing. During sleep the muscle tone becomes weaker, and the weight of flesh in the neck can cause the airway to collapse temporarily. This happens more often to people who are overweight. The severity of the problem varies widely—for some people it happens rarely. Even people with moderate to severe sleep apnea do not wake up every time their breathing stops, but the short interruption reduces the quality of their sleep and can lead them to feel tired even if they have slept all night.

If you suspect this may be the case, you should consult your doctor who can arrange for specific tests to be carried out. Equally, it is a good reason to lose a bit of weight.

How You Eat Determines How Well You Sleep

Many of the cycles of the body are controlled by hormones, which are chemical signals between the different parts of the brain and body. So it is not surprising to find that the chemicals we put into our body, in the form of food and drink, also have an effect on our sleep.

As we all differ from each other in a multitude of ways, there is a wide range of responses to the different chemicals, foods, and drinks we ingest. In order to make absolutely sure that you sleep well, we are going to remove all the potential sleep disruptors from your diet so that you are soon sleeping deeply.

Whenever we eat or drink something, parts of it are absorbed into our bloodstream and others are processed in the stomach and gut. So what we eat affects us in two ways—first via the chemicals that circulate swiftly through the body in the blood, and secondly via the nutrients released once digestion has started up and processed what we have consumed.

What Are the Best Foods to Help You Sleep?

Although we can think about going to sleep and can decide to go to bed when we feel tired, once we have given ourselves permission to sleep the process is overwhelmingly driven by neurochemicals and hormones. Chemicals that clash with the sleep hormones interfere with that process. If we take an "up" chemical when the body's cycle is trying to go down, there is a clash. This is what happens when we drink coffee—it contains caffeine that pushes the body towards alertness. In the morning that fits in nicely; late at night it sets up a fight with the rest of the body's chemical signals.

A healthy diet for sleep is actually very similar to a healthy diet for the waking portion of the day. Again, that is not surprising because sleep and wakefulness are two halves of a whole cycle. Your body has a natural intelligence. When you learn to listen carefully to that intelligence it will help you choose to eat the right amount of healthy food at the right time.

If your weight is fine but you just want to know what is best to eat to enhance your sleep, you don't need a lecture in nutrition. A simple rule is that fresh foods are better than processed foods. Many processed foods contain sugar, which gives you a rush when you eat them, overstimulating the body. Fresh foods have more fiber and are digested more easily, so you won't be kept awake by your stomach.

Once again, we find that diet is like exercise: what is good for maintaining fitness and a healthy weight is also good for your sleep. Eat healthily and use the strength and intelligence of your body during the day, and the natural cycle will help you sleep well at night.

The Magic Sleep Chemical Tryptophan

A lot of work has been done identifying foods that help you to fall asleep. Researchers have discovered that an amino acid called tryptophan helps you to sleep because when it is broken down it produces serotonin, which makes you feel good, and melatonin, which the body secretes to make you sleep as the light fades in the evening.

Tryptophan is common in turkey, so some people thought that eating turkey was especially good for promoting sleep. But actually there is tryptophan in milk and yogurt, in fish, in red meat, in all poultry, and in eggs. Many fruits, such as bananas and mangoes, contain tryptophan. In fact, it would be very difficult to avoid eating tryptophan in an ordinary diet. Pretty much any healthy diet will contain more than enough tryptophan to allow you to sleep well.

Indeed, any health diet must contain tryptophan because it is an "essential" amino acid. That means we need it, but our bodies do not synthesize it from other parts of our diet so we have to eat it.

Interestingly, tryptophan is common in chocolate, which also contains caffeine—which only goes to show that trying to control every single element of what you eat can get very, very complicated. It is far easier to learn to use your body's natural intelligence to guide you.

Timing

The time at which you eat can have a direct effect on your sleep. Specifically, it is important not to eat too much food too late at night. Digesting food is an active process. Blood is directed to the stomach and intestines, the stomach and the pancreas get to work, and the whole business takes time. If this is still happening while you are trying to get to sleep, it can feel uncomfortable. Furthermore, the digestive process works better when we are vertical (sitting or standing) than when we are lying down, simply because our stomach is above our intestines.

Another interesting research finding is that the energy from food eaten late at night is more likely to be turned into fat. The body has no immediate need for the amount of energy extracted from the food when you are about to fall asleep, so it stores it as fat, which is less likely to be used the next day than the energy from the food you eat then.

So simply:

Never eat later than three hours before going to sleep.

Don't eat too early or starve yourself either. Eat well enough so that your body has enough energy to let you sleep through till the morning.

What Are the Major Sleep-Disrupting Chemicals?

Caffeine

Caffeine is probably the most well-known chemical sleep disruptor. In many circumstances that is useful—people who want to stay focused or keep working late may take it to stay awake. It is well known that caffeine is present in coffee and in tea and in many "energy drinks," such as Red Bull or 5-Hour Energy. However, it is not so well known that caffeine is also present in many other drinks, such as colas, diet colas, and many other carbonated soft drinks. Even chocolate contains a small amount of caffeine. Many popular headache remedies contain caffeine because it helps the body to absorb the medication quicker.

The amount of caffeine in products varies widely. Instant coffee contains about as much caffeine as espresso coffee, but filter coffee contains at least half as much again. And it depends on which coffee beans you use. Robusta beans have twice as much caffeine as Arabica beans.

Tea contains caffeine, but tea bags tend to deliver more caffeine than loose-leaf tea, and leaving the tea to brew for five minutes instead of two almost doubles the amount of caffeine in the cup. All this shows how common caffeine is and how difficult it is to be accurate in measuring it.

Caffeine is metabolized in the body, and for normal, healthy adults it takes about three or four hours to remove half of it from the system and at least another three or four hours to remove the rest. So as you can see there are just too many variables to be precise about your caffeine intake. It is best to have no more than three cups of coffee per day, and even more importantly:

Don't consume caffeine after 2 P.M.

Interestingly, women taking the contraceptive pill take twice as long to metabolize caffeine, and pregnant women take twice as long as that, so they have to be even more careful.

Some people have a habit of drinking a lot of tea or coffee. They find that a cup of coffee perks them up—but then a couple of hours later they feel sleepy so they have another cup of coffee. And so it goes on. As they use coffee to stimulate themselves there is a "rebound" effect, and a few hours later they feel sleepy—more sleepy than they would have felt if they'd had no coffee at all. This can lead to taking "mini-naps" during the day, which can affect the longer sleep cycle.

If you drink a lot of coffee and find it makes you tired an hour or two later, try cutting down to no more than two cups—and the last one should be no later than after lunch.

The two rules of caffeine are simple:

1. Don't drink too much caffeine.

2. Never drink caffeine after 2 P.M.

Alcohol

Alcohol can cause or increase tiredness in the evening, but it has two negative effects on sleep. For each person the amount necessary to cause a negative effect varies—but typically it is well short of excessive drinking. The first negative effect is that it temporarily depresses the central nervous system, which causes the sleepiness, but which also leads to a "rebound" effect a few hours later. The second negative effect is that alcohol dehydrates the body. This is why many people can fall into a deep sleep after a few drinks, but then wake up in the middle of the night, thirsty and needing to go to the bathroom.

Even more alcohol takes them into hangover land with headaches and stomach upsets and all the other discomforts that affect sleep so badly.

The easiest way to be sure that alcohol is not contributing to your insomnia is to cut it out entirely. This will ensure you are able to establish a really robust pattern of deep sleep.

When your sleep has remained significantly better for several weeks, you can then, if you wish, try having an alcoholic drink and see if it has a negative effect. However, as with other potential sleep disruptors, it is important to test only one at a time so that you find out what your personal tolerances are. If you discover alcohol disrupts your sleep, you have found your limits. If not, you may find you can have a few drinks a few nights of the week.

However, it is not necessarily the case that you could drink the same amount every night, because the sleep cycle may be slightly affected and over several nights the effect could accumulate—to the extent that the cycle gets disrupted again. For most people it is a good idea to have a few days a week without alcohol to maintain a healthy cycle of deep sleep.

Other Drug Use

It will be no surprise to discover that research has demonstrated that many of the drugs people take for recreational purposes can have negative effects on sleep. Any drugs, legal or illegal, can affect sleep, so if you are in doubt, check with your doctor.

In a Nutshell

A vast amount of research has gone into the relationship between what we ingest and how we sleep, but it comes down to four simple rules:

EAT EARLY.

EAT HEALTHILY.

CUT OUT ALCOHOL AND THEN REINTRODUCE
IT ONLY IN MODERATION.

AVOID CAFFEINE.

• • •

CHAPTER 4

•

Your Sleep Environment

Your Sleep Environment

We all know people who can fall asleep almost anywhere—on the beach, in the sun, in a classroom, at the bus stop. I have a friend who even fell asleep at a rock concert. When your sleep cycle is robust and you are relaxed about it, you will find you can sleep in all sorts of circumstances. Many shift workers are able to do it. They just learn to adjust the start of their sleep to the hours they need. However, if your sleep cycle has been disrupted, you must make sure that the environment in which you sleep is as helpful as possible.

We're going to go through all the elements of your environment, so we can start restoring your sleep. Some of it may seem obvious, and in fact you may think you know some of it already—but please read the whole chapter carefully and follow the instructions because there may be some small, vital element that is new to you, and that might be the difference that makes all the difference.

The Power of Association

The human mind is very sensitive to associations. For example, whenever I go to the airport I get excited even if I am only dropping someone else off. I associate the airport with the excitement of travel. In the same way, nearly everyone has a favorite, comfortable chair where you sit down to relax. I have a sofa that is so easy to sink into that I relax as soon as I sit on it. I have to be really careful late at night that I don't fall asleep on it. In fact, I only have to think about lying on it and I can feel myself relaxing. This is the power of association!

When you remove the sleep disruptors in your life and create some positive sleep associations, everything begins changing. The first thing to do is to ensure that all the associations that influence you when you go to bed are ones that encourage sleep.

This is a vitally important part of the process. It is easy to forget how powerful our habits are because we are so very used to them—we stop noticing the things that we do every day because they are so familiar. However, there are a lot of things people do in bed because they can't sleep that just make things worse. I found out something fascinating when I worked with people who said they could not sleep.

For one reason or another, lots of them had developed a habit of reading in bed for an hour or more. Others went to bed, then got up again and went to the fridge and brought a snack back to bed. Others lay in bed and watched television.

They had all gotten into the habit of doing these different things in bed that were keeping them awake, so they had accidentally taught themselves to be insomniacs! They had associated things that kept them awake with the place where they were trying to sleep.

It is essential that you break any associations that are keeping you awake. From now on, it is vital that you stick to this rule.

There are only three things you ever do in bed:

1. Sleep.

2. Make love.

3. Read this book or listen to the hypnotic trance.

This means no TV, no eating, and no reading novels till late into the night. If you have a TV in your bedroom, take it out. If you can't take it out of the bedroom, pull out the plug so you are not tempted to flick it on. And turn your alarm clock away from you so you cannot see it. Lots of people who have insomnia keep opening their eyes and looking at the time. As you learn to sleep better that is another habit to change. Your alarm will wake you up in the morning; you don't need to look at it all night long. This may sound a bit simplistic, but you will discover pretty soon that associations are very powerful indeed.

There is one more rule that follows from number 3 above:

4. If you are awake in bed for more than 20 minutes, you must do one of the exercises (see the index on page 144) or get up and do something boring.

We are building the association between bed and sleep, so if you are not sleeping, making love, or using this book or the hypnotic trance, you shouldn't be in bed. Go back to bed only when you feel sleepy again.

Some people ask me if all this is really necessary— and the answer is: "Yes!"

Association is a powerful force so it is vital that you do not give any more power to the old association of poor sleep in your bed.

When you do this, the power of association begins to work for you. The unconscious mind is particularly sensitive to association and will increasingly associate bed with sleep. When you really follow these rules properly, you will find that your sleep improves rapidly.

How the Amount of Light and Dark Affects Your Sleep

Our bodies have a mechanism that adjusts our sleepiness to the hours of darkness. A part of the brain called the hypothalamus is connected to the back of the eyes and, according to the amount of light it perceives, it releases different hormones: cortisol, which wakes us up in the morning, or melatonin, which sends us to sleep at night.

Because this natural system is hardwired into our brains, light can have a very strong effect on us. That's why we have another simple but important rule:

Keep your bedroom really dark at night.

In the summer it can still be quite light some time after you wish to go to bed, and in the winter there is so much street lighting that many houses are bathed in light even in the middle of the night. So a simple but vital preparation for good sleep is to ensure you have curtains or blinds that truly keep out the light. If your curtains are made of a light material, you can line them or just buy a dark blind to hang behind them covering the window. Alternatively, you can use an eye mask, like the ones you get on airplanes.

Of course, when you are tired it is possible to sleep even when it's bright daylight, but if you make your sleeping environment properly dark, then you are getting one more part of the environment on your side. As it is so easy and practical, you might as well do it.

Sleeping Soundly

It's amazing how your brain can make noise unimportant. When I moved to New York in the mid-1990s, the first night I wondered how I was ever going to get to sleep with the constant traffic and sirens wailing all night long. Within a few nights I wasn't even aware of the noise outside. I only became aware of the sounds when other people from out of town came over and mentioned the noise and I found myself aware of it again. This is because of a simple psychological principle: the conscious mind is always looking for novelty. It's part of our self-protection mechanism, to search for anything that's different in case it's a threat. After a while, when we realize it's not a threat, the mind learns to ignore it. That means that however noisy it is, when our minds get used to the noise we can easily fall asleep because:

**The mind learns to ignore
unimportant stimulus.**

This is how people are able to live next door to a railway track and after a few days not even notice it. If your area is simply noisy all the time, it is unlikely that you need to do anything about it. As your mind gets used to hearing repeated noises, after a while it will ignore them and you will sleep perfectly.

The sort of noises that wake us at night are those that are variable and intermittent, or that catch our attention, such as TV or radio dialogue. So to stack the cards in your favor:

Reduce your exposure to variable noise.

Sometimes just reducing the volume is all that is necessary. You can do that by using earplugs. Alternatively, you can mask external noises by playing a recording of natural sounds like waves, waterfalls, or forest noise. But if you want to listen to anything, the best place to start is to listen to the hypnotic trance.

Incidentally, the hypnotic trance also contains special suggestions that will help your mind to integrate any distracting noises into your system of falling asleep.

How Simple Physical Comfort Can Enhance Your Sleep

For some people the only solution required to restore their sleep cycle is ridiculously simple:

Make sure your bed is comfortable.

Many people keep their mattresses, pillows, or duvets for far too long. All of them get worn out eventually, and they become less and less comfortable. It is a terrible thing to go to bed and not even feel comfortable.

So just check: if you are at home now, go and check the pillows, the duvet or blankets, and the mattress. Think about it this way. If you checked into a luxury hotel for a weekend, would you be happy to sleep in the bed you see now? Most people can only afford a night in a luxury hotel on very special occasions—but you sleep in your own bed almost every night. It is much better value to spend the money on your own bed than blow it on one extravagant night, even if you do have to save up for a while. You can even get a mattress topper, which can transform a bed that has seen better days. There's an old saying that still holds true. "Never skimp on your bed or shoes, because if you are not in one, you are in the other."

Temperature

Research has shown that we sleep best when we are comfortably warm in bed and the air in the room is cool. If the room is too hot, we tend to wake up too easily. It is a very simple matter to check that you turn down the heating or the radiators in your room. Some people—but not all—find that it is also helpful to have their feet slightly cooler than the rest of their bodies. To find out if you are such a person, try sticking your feet out of the bed, or have them covered by just a sheet.

It is just as important to check that you are not too cold in bed. As duvets get older they become less efficient, so you may need to buy a new one or put a blanket or rug on top. During the night your body temperature gradually falls, and it is at its lowest around three or four in the morning. You need to make sure that your bedding is warm enough to keep you comfortable then. I have found quite a few people who were waking up in the middle of the night just because they were a fraction too cold. As soon as they used a warmer blanket or duvet they slept all the way through the night.

Remember the air in the bedroom should still be cooler than your bed so don't turn up the heating too high—just make sure that your blankets or duvet are warm enough.

Keep warm in bed in a cool room.

Allergies

Some people are prone to allergies and have a mild allergic reaction to their pillows or to the detergents they use on their bed linen. It may not cause discomfort, but it is just enough to wake them during the night.

This is extremely rare, but it is easy to test. Use a different laundry detergent or try a different pillow. If you find your sleep improves dramatically, keep using the new detergent or the new pillow.

Play the Hypnotic Trance

If you are concerned there could be some noise when you go to bed, play the hypnotic trance. The dialogue and soundtrack are specifically designed to help you sleep, and it will also neatly mask any other noises outside your bedroom. Those noises are still there, of course, but they are moved to the background of your awareness, so that while you fall asleep your conscious awareness can hear my words and the background soundtrack blends in to all the other sounds to promote a relaxed response in the brain.

In a Nutshell

MAKE SURE THE BEDROOM IS
DARK, COOL, AND QUIET.

MAKE SURE YOUR BED IS
WARM AND COMFORTABLE.

ONLY SLEEP, MAKE LOVE, OR USE THIS
BOOK AND HYPNOTIC TRANCE IN BED.

• • •

•

CHAPTER 5

Running Your Own Mind

Running Your Own Mind

People work to make their homes nice, to go on vacation, and to buy things to make themselves feel good. However, the majority of people spend almost no time directly changing how they think and feel. They leave it to chance and hope they feel good. But we create an inner world with our imagination, our memories, and our internal dialogue and it can have just as much impact on us as the outside world. In this chapter we are going to learn how to change that inner world and use it to significantly improve your sleep.

Many people who can't sleep have accidentally created patterns of thinking that keep them awake. For example, far too many people spend too much time thinking about all the things that could go wrong for them. They worry about all the possible problems and go over them again and again. The irony is that they stay awake, and because they are tired they are less able to deal with their concerns.

Some worrying is useful. It's good to think about possible problems so that you can work out how to address them. We need to be prepared. However, far too many people only think about what could go wrong and forget to think about what could go right.

Whatever you focus on sends a message to the mind that says, "This is how I want events to go." It becomes a self-fulfilling prophecy. So as well as worries, we need to have solutions. Of course, we can't always find the solution right away with our conscious mind, so I'm also going to show you an amazing way of using your unconscious mind to help you.

Using Your Whole Mind

You may remember earlier I referred to the two parts of the mind, the conscious and the unconscious minds. The **conscious mind** is the part with which you actively think and make decisions and with which you are reading this book right now. In the **unconscious mind** you store your memories, learning, and habits and the automatic behaviors that you use every day to run your life. It also contains all the "hardwired" aspects of you that run the basic functions of your body. It keeps your heart beating and your lungs breathing, and it also organizes the patterns of your sleep.

Going to sleep requires cooperation between the conscious and unconscious minds. Your unconscious sends to your conscious mind a signal that it is time to sleep by making you feel tired and sleepy. As we saw earlier, there is no point at all in going to bed until you get that signal. Then when you do really feel tired and sleepy, you use your conscious mind to check there is no overriding need to stay awake. If it is safe to go to sleep, you simply agree with your unconscious mind to let it happen, and you hand over to the unconscious to run the sleep program. The unconscious mind makes sleep happen by changing your body chemistry, creating muscular relaxation, and slowing the thoughts of your mind so that you drift into a different state of consciousness.

I have had some people come to me with sleeping problems who say, "I want to go to sleep, but when I go to bed I just can't stop my brain from working." What they don't realize is the brain should always be working. It is keeping you alive and healthy. The point is not to "stop your brain from working" but to let the unconscious mind carry on working while your conscious mind goes to sleep. In this chapter I will show you how to do that. We will reinstall the habits of the unconscious mind that help you go to sleep smoothly and stay as deeply asleep as you need, and I will also show you how to prepare your conscious mind to help you feel more comfortable, more relaxed, and more sleepy.

What Are You Putting into Your Mind?

Just as it is helpful to get your physical environment right to help you sleep, the psychological environment of your mind needs to be right as well.

Everything you perceive causes your body to react. For example, if you witnessed a terrible car crash you would have a strong reaction. Your body would automatically see the crash as dangerous and trigger the "fight or flight" response.

This is our self-protection mechanism and dates back to when we were cave-dwellers and our survival depended on being able to fight an enemy or run away. Adrenaline is released into the bloodstream, blood is pumped to the major muscles, the heartbeat quickens, the digestive system stops, the immune system is suppressed, and our muscles tense up.

It is a fascinating and important fact that when you are engrossed in a film or even vividly imagining an event the human nervous system has the same kind of response as it does to a real event. For example, if you see a realistic film of a dangerous situation, your body tenses up. That is why you find yourself gasping or gripping your seat when watching an action movie or a horror film.

Of course, films like that are entertainment, but for some people they can contribute to their trouble with sleeping. If your body is reacting to shock and excitement, it releases stress chemicals, and for some people that is just too much stimulation in the hour before going to bed.

So there is a simple way to make sure you establish a really solid pattern of deep sleep. We need to make sure you don't wind yourself up when you need to wind down.

It is not just action movies that keep you alert. All television programs are designed to catch your attention and to keep it by making you excited. TV is designed to do the opposite of send you to sleep because the program makers want you to keep watching, to see all the commercials. Even everyday programs like the news focus on shocking and unusual events. People having a nice, happy time do not make for very exciting news, so the bulletins are full of crashes, floods, explosions, financial problems, and lucky escapes.

Of course, there are some people who have no trouble at all in watching disaster reports, thrillers, dramas, and horror movies and then sleeping very well. However, if you are having trouble sleeping, don't let the TV keep you awake. Therefore, while you are reestablishing a solid pattern of sleep:

**Switch off the TV at least one hour
before you go to bed.**

This gives your mind a chance to process and absorb all the adrenaline released in response to the exciting imagery, to slow down to a more gentle pace that will synchronize with your natural impetus towards sleep.

The Movies of Your Mind

TV is not the only source of pictures that we react to. We also make pictures in our minds as we think and remember and imagine things.

This process is called visualization. Some people tell me they don't believe they can visualize—but I have not yet met anyone who can't do it. Let me show you what I mean by visualization. I'm going to ask you a couple of questions.

What color is the front door of your home?

Which side is the lock on?

In order to answer these questions you had to go into your memory and make an image. You "saw" your front door and thought of the right name for the color. You may even have imagined opening the door in order to remember which side the lock is on.

Here's another example.

Think of a good holiday you had, and now choose one particular time and place where you really enjoyed yourself. Bring it to mind nice and clearly, and now answer this question:

What was the weather like?

To answer that question you had to see that specific time and place in your mind's eye and remember whether it was sunny or not.

To answer the questions about your front door and about the holiday weather you created images in your mind. That is visualization. Of course, these images will not be "photo quality"—and that's a good thing.

You need to be able to tell the difference between the real world and your imagination. We use these images, in much the same way as we use our internal voice, to think about things. And researchers have found out that how we use these pictures has a significant effect on how we feel.

The human nervous system cannot tell the difference between a real and a vividly imagined event. So when people lie in bed at night imagining pictures of events that make them feel anxious it is not just their ideas that are affected—the whole of their body experiences the stressful chemicals that are released. These internal pictures and movies can keep them awake. In fact, working with insomniacs I found that most of them were making pictures during the day of themselves lying awake at night in their beds. They were running the movies over and over again in their minds and producing stress chemicals in their bodies. They were keeping themselves awake just by imagining being kept awake.

The fact that they managed to keep themselves awake by imagining staying awake shows just how easy it is to program the mind. We are going to use that same ability to program your mind to go to sleep.

Reducing Your Worries

Read this exercise through carefully before you do it.

1. Remember now one of the things you lay
    awake and worried about. Bring it to mind
    and picture it now. It may be something
    from the past that still worried you, or
    something you were worrying about in the
    future such as not being able to sleep. You
    may see it as a few pictures—for example,
    someone's face or a room full of people—or
    you may see it as a sort of mini-video, a film
    of something happening or people watching
    you and talking. It doesn't matter what sort
    of picture or video it is—just see it in your
    mind however it looks to you.

2. Next, step out of the image like a special
    effect in a movie—in other words, imagine
    floating out of yourself, so that you can see
    the back of your head as you float farther
    and farther away until you can see yourself
    in the picture.

3. Now float the image away from you another
    12 feet so that you can see the stressful situ-
    ation as if it's happening to someone else.

4. Next drain out all the color from the image until it's only in black and white like a very old movie.

5. Now shrink it down in size until it's a lot smaller.

6. Keep watching it and make it as transparent as you can.

7. Finally, now that the emotional intensity has been reduced, ask yourself if you need to make any decisions about the situation, and if you do, make those decisions using the calmness and sense of distance you have now that you can see the situation like this.

To be guided through this process, play the video "Calm the Images in Your Mind."

Feeling Drowsy

Now that you have reduced your worries, let me show you a very, very simple exercise that will help you get ready to sleep and that also shows just how powerful pictures can be. I am indebted to my good friend Richard Bandler for this simple and elegant idea.

Practicing Being Drowsy

Read this exercise through carefully before you do it—and don't do this unless you are ready to go to sleep.

1. Remember a time when you felt very tired, and remember how your body felt.

2. Now, keeping that feeling, imagine you are surrounded by some of your friends who are all just as tired as you.

3. As you look around, notice that one of them yawns. Watch them yawn. Then another one yawns.

4. As more people begin to yawn, notice how you feel, and notice that some people are having difficulty keeping their eyes open.

5. And let yourself join in the yawning.

6. Notice whether your eyes want to close, and even if your eyes are already closed, imagine them closing again, imagine them flickering then closing again, over and over again.

7. Yawn again and notice where you feel the yawn—in your throat or jaw—and let your mind drift, and every time you find yourself drifting back again, just look around again at the circle of tired, yawning people.

8. As you yawn more, notice a warm, comfortable feeling spreading around you, and let yourself drift again.

• • •

CHAPTER 6

•

The Power of Your Internal Voice

The Power of Your Internal Voice

As well as pictures, we all use an "internal voice" as part of our thinking. We use this voice when we are making decisions and reflecting and commenting on things. Whether we are aware of it or not, we are using it most of the time we are awake. For example, you might be going shopping and say to yourself, "I must remember to buy some more bread." Or before you ask someone a question, you rehearse it in your mind before you speak it out loud. Mostly we use our internal voice to comment on what's happening in the world around us.

One particular aspect of this internal voice is very, very important to us because researchers have found that the way we talk to ourselves has a significant effect on how we feel. For example, pay attention to your internal voice right now. Say something to yourself about sleep. Now, stop and notice where that voice is located. Is it at the front of your head, the back, or to the side? Just check now—does it seem to be inside your head or outside? If it is in your head, is it to the front of your head or the back? Is it higher up or lower down?

Now that you have established where it is, say that phrase to yourself again. This time, notice the tone of the internal voice. Is it chatty? Anxious? Authoritative? Friendly? Is it excited or sad or neutral?

Researchers have found that the tone of our internal voice affects how we feel—but crucially, most of the time we don't think about it and simply let the world around us determine the tone of voice we use. So if we feel we are in a stressful situation, we tend to speak to ourselves with a sense of urgency; if it is a frustrating situation, we tend to use an irritated tone; if it's a relaxing situation, we tend to have a relaxed tone.

However, it is the tone of voice more than the situation that determines how you feel. So if you make a mistake and tell yourself off with a voice like an old schoolteacher, your tone makes you feel bad. If you are nice to yourself and use a sweet, seductive tone of voice, you will instantly feel better.

The amazing thing is that you can simply choose to change the tone of the internal voice and it automatically changes how you feel. Try this as an experiment.

Remember a time you really made a mistake and how you criticized yourself. What kind of things did you say to yourself?

Next, remember those harsh critical statements.

However, now make the tone of them sexy. Imagine how it would sound if you criticized yourself in a seductive, sexy voice. Try it now and notice how difficult it is to feel as stressed as you did when the tone of voice was harsh and critical.

Learning to change the tone of the internal voice is a vital part of learning to run your own mind, and it is immensely useful in learning to promote regular, restful sleep. I have found lots of insomniacs who lay in bed and talked to themselves about not sleeping, but what's really interesting is that they did it in a tone of voice that was actually helping to keep them awake. When I examined closely exactly how they were talking to themselves I found they were all using some version of an irritated, frustrated, or in some way agitated tone of voice. The pace was also fast. The result was that feelings of irritation or agitation kept them in a physiological state of excitement, which kept them awake.

Shortly we are going to practice changing the tone of your internal voice and you will gain more mastery over how you feel. As you become good at it you will be able to send yourself to sleep by making your internal dialogue slow and sleepy sounding.

You know how certain tones of voice make you feel sleepy. We've all met boring people who drone on and on until you find your mind drifting and feel unable to stay awake. Or when you think about the tone of voice you would use to tell a bedtime story, it starts to make you relax.

One of the most important parts of this system is to learn to use your internal voice to work for you. A great way to do this is to make your internal voice speak at a very slow pace in a tired, gentle tone of voice. I teach people to use this slow, gentle tone of voice when I am teaching them self-hypnosis because relaxation is a key part and this calming, gentle voice automatically evokes a relaxation response in the body. That is why hypnotists use a monotonous, slow tone of voice, and mothers naturally speak in a gentle, relaxing tone of voice when they are lulling their babies to sleep. You can use the same technique now.

Calming the Internal Voice

Read this exercise through carefully before you do it. Although the technique is simple, it is worth getting every part of it right so that it works really well.

1. Remember something you used to say as you lay awake at night, for example, "This is so boring, I can't sleep. I don't know how I'll cope tomorrow. Oh, if only I could sleep." And so on.

2. Say it all again to yourself now, and notice where the voice is located. To the front of your head, the back, or is it outside?

3. Now repeat the same phrase. Move the voice a little farther away, imagine how it would sound as it moves off into the distance.

4. Now notice the tone of the internal voice. Is it frustrated? Is it angry? Is it depressed? Whatever it was, change the tone so that the voice sounds happily tired and drowsy—as though the voice can hardly stay awake. Say exactly the same words again in a really drowsy, relaxed voice. And notice, again, how different you feel.

5. Finally repeat the same words with that happy, drowsy, tired tone of voice and this time, let the voice yawn in between the words. So that (yawn) every few words (yawn) the voice has to stop to (yawn and yawn), and you notice how very delightfully, comfortably tired you feel as you hear those words (yawn) drifting around your awareness.

6. In future, practice this talking to yourself in a slow, drowsy, yawning voice for several minutes before you go to bed.

For more practice, play the video "Calm Your Internal Dialogue."

Drowsy Associations

The legendary hypnotist Milton Erickson was famous for being able to hypnotize anyone. While Milton was eloquent in his use of hypnotic language, he would often talk in a slow, quiet, rhythmic, monotone voice for hours at a time. Many psychologists tried to study Erickson, but couldn't stay awake as they sat there for hours listening and watching him work with a client.

In fact, after he had hypnotized a client several times, their mind made the association between deep relaxation and the particular tone of voice Milton used when he put them into a trance. So Milton would only have to use that slow, rhythmic, monotonous voice and you couldn't stay awake.

Getting good at getting drowsy is just like any skill, like riding a bike or playing the guitar—the more you practice it, the better at it you get.

You have practiced how to stay awake by describing to yourself during the day how you were going to be wide awake and unable to sleep at night, and you did it over and over again until it became a self-fulfilling prophecy.

Before going to sleep spend ten minutes talking to yourself in a slow monotonous voice and practice making yourself drowsy.

Do it for ten minutes now—speak to yourself about anything, it could be your shopping list, but do it with a monotonous, yawning internal voice and make yourself drowsy. Drone on and on until you feel sleepy. After a while you will only have to talk in this drowsy tone of voice and you will begin to feel sleepy.

Using the Internal Voice to Put You to Sleep

This process is used by hypnotists, meditators, and doctors the world over to help people calm their minds and bodies. It is very simple, but like anything, the more you practice the better you get.

It simply involves thinking about a particular area of your body and relaxing it. Some people like to tell themselves silently in their heads: "Now I am relaxing my shoulders."

Systematic Relaxation

Read through this exercise first before you do it, and remember: only do it where you can safely relax completely, such as in bed.

1. Use your most comfortable, tired, drowsy voice and simply say each of the following to yourself as you do it.

    Now I relax my eyes

    Now I relax my jaw

    Now I relax my tongue

    Now I relax my shoulders

    Now I relax my arms

Now I relax my hands

Now I relax my chest

Now I relax my stomach

Now I relax my thighs

Now I relax my calves

Now I relax my feet

Now I relax my mind

2. At this point you may find it helpful to go through the whole process again several times to deepen the relaxation.

Like every other skill you learn in life, this gets easier, and you get better at it, with practice. So every night practice speaking to yourself with a contented, happy, tired, drowsy voice that yawns, so that it becomes a natural, automatic part of falling asleep easily.

What's Your Story?

In our society people are labeled far too much. For example, children are told they are hyperactive, or they are labeled as either sporty or academic. If the label is repeated, people take it on as an identity and build stories to support it.

Some stories are positive: "I'm good at math," or "I'm a loyal friend." Others are negative: "I'm no good in social situations," or "I'm a poor sleeper."

And while there may be some truth in these stories, the more we tell ourselves these stories, the more we believe them. They are all just stories. Some of them support us and some of them don't. But they can be changed. Over the years I have seen so many people change. In particular, I have seen a lot of people who had been told they were "incurable" get better.

Back in the 1950s a young singer played his first gig in Nashville, Tennessee. When he came off stage, the manager of the venue said to him, "You ain't going nowhere, son. You ought to go back to driving a truck."

In the 1970s a couple of students went to the big computer companies with the new, small computer they'd built and asked for a job. They were told that they weren't needed. If they had given up at that point, Steve Jobs and Steve Wozniak would never have started Apple Computer. And if that young singer had just gone back to driving a truck, the world would never have heard of Elvis Presley. They succeeded because they did not accept the label someone else offered them.

Sometimes we take a label and apply it to ourselves. In a way, that can be more of a problem because we get used to it and take it for granted in all the stories we tell ourselves.

A lot of people who have come to me with sleep issues begin by telling me their story about why they are different and can't change. Sometimes it almost feels as though they have been brainwashed. These are some of the things they were saying to themselves:

- *I've always been an insomniac, I've never slept well.*

- *I'm different from everyone else.*

- *I can't change, insomnia runs in the family.*

- *I've been doing this so long nothing is going to change it.*

- *I don't think it was the pictures that kept me awake.*

- *My worries are far too real.*

- *Whatever I do won't make any difference.*

What these people haven't yet realized is that that same story they are eager for me to believe is exactly what's holding them back from the changes they want to make.

I was working recently with someone who said to me, "I just can't sleep, I'm an insomniac."

"That's what you tell yourself?" I replied.

"No, no," he said, "you don't understand, I really am an insomniac."

"That's what you tell yourself?" I said again.

We repeated this little exchange three or four times before he could actually hear the question I was asking him. "You're right," he said, somewhat astonished, "that is what I'm telling myself."

"So now," I asked him, "are you ready to tell yourself something different?"

Saying "I'm an insomniac" is defining yourself by your past. That's like saying, "I can't run, because I'm a person who stands still." If you define yourself by what you have done in the past, you will repeat the past. If you define yourself as someone who is free to make choices in the present, you can change your future. What you've said about yourself in the past is a story you tell yourself. You can change the story you tell yourself.

I'm now going to show you how to let go, stage by stage, of any old stories about insomnia so that your natural sleep cycle can return.

Changing Your Story

Read this exercise through carefully before you do it.

1. Think of a time in the past when you were telling yourself that you couldn't sleep. Remember it like you are back there again now. What did you say to yourself? For

example: "I can't sleep." "There's nothing I can do, it's happening again." "I can't change, it runs in the family." It doesn't matter if you can't remember the exact words, just the sense of it. Hear that internal voice and notice where it is.

2. Now, just as in the exercise on page 77, imagine stepping out of yourself like a special effect in a movie so that you can see yourself in that situation as if it was happening to someone else.

3. Watch yourself over there talking to yourself and imagine you can overhear what you are saying to yourself over there, 12 feet away from you.

4. As you hear that old story from 12 feet away, notice how different it feels to hear it like that.

5. Now turn down the volume of that story over there.

6. And over here, choose how you are going to describe yourself as a good sleeper—for example, "I'm sleeping better and better," "I sleep so deeply now," or "I've discovered how to get to sleep anywhere."

When you hear that voice over there, it means there is room for a different story over here. As you experiment with different ways of describing your success, you will change for the better the unconscious assumptions you used to make about sleep.

• • •

CHAPTER 7

•

What to Do When Your Head Fills with Thoughts

What to Do When Your Head Fills with Thoughts

Quite often our lives get filled up with relatively unimportant things and it is difficult to find enough time for yourself. The only time you get to think things over is right at the very end of the day when you have some time to yourself, in bed, in the dark and quiet, so the unconscious seizes the moment just before you go to sleep to get you to think about what really matters to you. That is actually a good thing—it is just not the most convenient time to do it.

So what you need to do is to take that time for yourself—but to shift it to a more convenient time of day. Set aside at least 20 minutes to think about your own priorities and to work out a way to achieve them.

If you have been kept awake by a busy mind, do this every day for at least three weeks. It is a good habit to have anyway, but after a while you may find that if you are not too busy you need to do it only once or twice a week. If your life gets busy again, you may have to do it every day.

Value Yourself

Read this exercise through carefully before you do it.

1. Find yourself a time and place where you can be undisturbed for 20 minutes. Take a pad of paper and a pen.

2. For the first five minutes let your mind wan-
    der and think about anything under the sun.

3. After five minutes, ask yourself this question:
    "What do I want to do that is really impor-
    tant to me?" Make a note of everything that
    comes to mind. Don't censor it or order or
    rank it, just write down absolutely everything
    whether it seems important or ridiculous,
    everyday or fantastic. You can include any-
    thing. For example, you could want to move
    house, learn to dance, write a book, get
    married, visit the pyramids, buy some new
    shoes, or change your job.

4. When you feel you're done, just reread the
    list slowly and add on anything else that
    comes to mind while you are reading it.

5. Now—and only now—go over the list one
    more time and divide the items into two
    groups—"important to have" and just "nice
    to have."

6. Now choose one of the "important to have"
    items and ask yourself this question: "What
    is the smallest, practical, achievable step I
    can take tomorrow that will move me to-
    wards reaching this goal?"

7. Think about it, make sure that your step is realistic and sensible and commit yourself to taking that step tomorrow. It could be a very small step—just making one phone call or looking up one piece of information on the Internet, but whatever it is, make a solemn promise to yourself to take that step.

Do this exercise as often as you need to and you will create two successful achievements:

1. You will sleep better and better.

2. You will move, step by step, towards getting what really matters to you.

Number 2 is a great side effect! You won't be lying there thinking, "What if?" Instead you can go to sleep knowing that tomorrow you will get another step closer to your goals.

Emotional Intelligence

We've looked at how to get your mind to start converting your worries into a plan for action. With a bit of time and reflection and using the exercises I've shown you, you can get a sense of proportion about problems and challenges, and a lot of little difficulties just melt away. All that means that you really can drift off to sleep without being stopped by needless distractions, but sometimes there are things that seem stubborn. They won't stop nagging you.

What do we do about feelings and ideas that just won't go away? Apart from the stuff we've now dealt with, there are two sorts of things that keep your mind busy: inspiration and emotions.

Inspiration

Sometimes we don't sleep because we suddenly have a great idea. It might be irritating that you have your flash of inspiration just as you want to go to sleep, but there is a reason why ideas come at that time. Life can be busy, so you don't always have time to get in touch with your creativity, so when you have a bit of peace and quiet and there is nothing urgent to do, your unconscious mind takes the chance to present you with the results of your creative potential.

There is a very simple way to deal with this.

**Keep pen and paper by your bed and
write down your inspiration.**

Once you've made your notes or sketch, you can relax knowing your idea won't be lost if you forget it. It is not just great artists who have great ideas. Of course, it is not the case that every flash of inspiration is as brilliant the next day as you thought it was the night before, but sometimes those ideas contain the seeds of brilliance.

It's almost like making an agreement with your unconscious mind. If you make a note of it, you are more likely to take action so your mind won't need to wake you.

Emotions

We have already seen how to get worries in perspective with the exercise in the previous chapter. Sometimes, if the feeling was just caused by the way you were seeing things in your mind, it disappears when you get it in perspective. But other times it doesn't disappear, it stays with you. If an emotion doesn't go away when you change the pictures in your mind, it means it is an emotion that carries an important message for you.

Emotions are another part of our intelligence, and we need to pay attention to them in order to learn more about ourselves and how we are getting on in the world. That doesn't mean we have to react—it means we have to listen to their message. Here's a simple but very powerful way to understand your emotions, which will help you to sleep.

Life throws us many challenges and some of them give rise to strong emotions. Whatever you are facing, it is helpful to be able to be calm and to learn from your emotions. This exercise will let you understand your feelings better so that you have a clearer idea of what you need to do.

It is impossible to live without some fear because it is a natural part of our defenses. Emotions are signals. They say, "Pay attention to this." We want some fear if we are about to step off the curb without looking, to make us pay attention to the traffic to stop us getting run over. We want some anger if someone is mean to us, so we can stand up for ourselves. If I have done something wrong to my friend, I want some guilt because it motivates me to repair the relationship. Emotions are our friends. However, because some of them feel uncomfortable we are often taught to ignore them. Some people go out and get drunk or overeat or bury themselves in work to avoid their emotions. The more they do this, the more the emotion shouts. And what is the best time for an emotion to catch your attention? In that gap between waking and sleep when you are naturally clearing your mind of all the concerns of the day. What is quite miraculous, though, is that as soon as you listen to an emotion it delivers its message and it disappears. This doesn't mean that everything you feel is meaningful. Phobias, for example, are feelings that are shouting too loud too often.

However, generally we do have the chance to benefit from the wisdom of our emotions, and that is what we are about to do.

The exercise below works with any strong emotion that is nagging you when you want to sleep. You'll see that I start by saying "feel the emotion." At first that sounds silly—after all, if you weren't already feeling the emotion, there wouldn't be a problem in the first place. But the point is just to feel it without any reaction or judgment. That sounds simple, and it is, but it requires just a little patience to let yourself simply feel the emotion and stay with it without doing anything or reacting. You will soon get the hang of it. In the hypnotic trance we will make this easier by inviting your unconscious mind to recalibrate your emotions so that you can more easily receive the message of your emotions without overwhelm.

Here is an example of how it works.

I worked with a businessman who knew immediately exactly how he felt. I'd hardly had a chance to ask him when he said, "Angry."

I asked him why he was angry, and he told me that the people he was dealing with had lied to him. Then I asked him to bear with me and answer a question that might seem a bit obvious. I asked him, "Why does that matter to you?" He replied he felt they were patronizing him. Again I asked, "Why does that matter to you?"

"Because I don't feel like I'm being heard," he replied. I asked my question yet again and he said, "It matters because I want to be treated with respect."

Then he looked quite surprised and said to me, "I feel much calmer."

The reason he felt calmer was because he had moved from being angry with something to recognizing the positive value that his anger was defending.

He knew what he needed to do was to make sure that the people who had angered him treated him with respect.

The purpose of his anger was to defend his self-respect. His emotion was telling him to stand up for himself. Now that he had received the message from his emotions, he knew he could be angry if necessary, but it was no longer overwhelming him. Furthermore, he could also do other things to ensure that he received the right amount of respect.

The same procedure works with any emotion. For example, another client said that she lay in bed at night and couldn't stop feeling anxious. I asked her to feel the anxiety again and to ask herself, "Why am I anxious?"

Her first reply was a long list of worries about her children, her partner, and her parents. At the end, I simply asked, "Why does that matter to you?" She said she cared about them all but was worried for them. I asked, "Why does that matter to you?" again and again and again, and then she said, "Because I love them all." When she said that, she suddenly realized that behind her anxiety was all the love and affection and joy that she got from her family. Her anxiety was simply trying to get her to acknowledge and enjoy all those wonderful feelings.

If you have a nagging feeling that won't go away, use the following exercise.

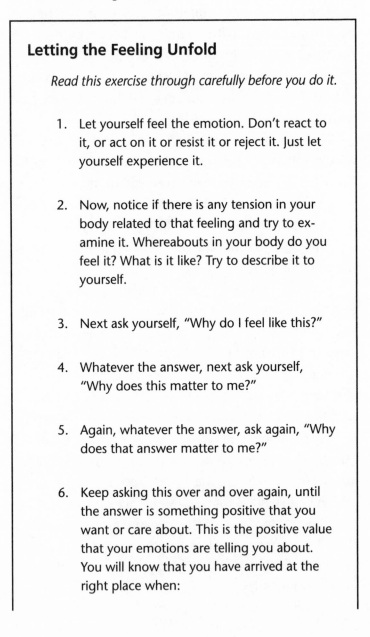

Letting the Feeling Unfold

Read this exercise through carefully before you do it.

1. Let yourself feel the emotion. Don't react to it, or act on it or resist it or reject it. Just let yourself experience it.

2. Now, notice if there is any tension in your body related to that feeling and try to examine it. Whereabouts in your body do you feel it? What is it like? Try to describe it to yourself.

3. Next ask yourself, "Why do I feel like this?"

4. Whatever the answer, next ask yourself, "Why does this matter to me?"

5. Again, whatever the answer, ask again, "Why does that answer matter to me?"

6. Keep asking this over and over again, until the answer is something positive that you want or care about. This is the positive value that your emotions are telling you about. You will know that you have arrived at the right place when:

> - *It is a positive feeling—something you wish for, not something you reject.*
>
> - *It is personal—it is about your values, not about what anyone else thinks, does, or feels.*
>
> - *The original feeling is noticeably reduced or changed.*
>
> 7. Pay attention to this positive, personal feeling and you will notice now that your original feeling has been transformed into something positive and motivating.

When you use this exercise you will find that disturbing emotions are actually reminding you of what matters to you most. When you know what that is, it is easier to be much clearer about what you really want in the future. When you are clear about the positives in your life, it is easier to relax, and you find you can drift easily and comfortably off to sleep.

Of course, there can be many levels to our ambitions. We all have a lot to learn from our emotions, and it can take time and effort to make our ambitions come true. And sometimes we just don't know how we are going to do it. If you really don't know how you are going to reach your goals, the next exercise is for you.

Asking the Unconscious Mind to Help

When I talked to people who thought they were insomniacs, I noticed that almost all of them talked to themselves about being awake when they lay in bed. The longer they lay awake at night, the more they talked about being awake. Some of them would imagine hours of sleeplessness ahead, some would make pictures of being overtired the next day, others would ask themselves why they weren't sleeping and think of all the different things that could have caused them to stay awake. All this thinking and talking was focused on one thing—being awake!

This reminded me of a pattern I had seen elsewhere. People on diets think about all the food they are not eating, smokers who are unsuccessful at quitting think about cigarettes they are missing—and insomniacs think about how much they are going to stay awake at night. They all had one thing in common: they were all focusing on the problem, not on the solution. One of the most important practical rules of psychology that has helped me achieve consistently good results over the years is this:

**You always get more of
what you focus on.**

This is because the unconscious mind is monitoring everything we think about, so when people feed themselves images of staying awake, the unconscious mind takes that as a command and helps to do more of it.

This is called a negative feedback loop. Focusing on what you don't want produces more of what you don't want. In fact, I found that a large number of the people I helped had no other problem than this. As soon as they learned to focus on sleep and not wakefulness, their sleep improved dramatically overnight.

On the other hand, using hypnosis both with clients and for myself I have been amazed at the creativity and resourcefulness of the unconscious mind. Over and over again I have witnessed people calling on the help and wisdom of the unconscious and making things happen that seemed almost miraculous. But as well as hypnosis there is another, older way to utilize the power of the unconscious, which is to activate it during our sleep. We can simply ask the unconscious to work for us while we are sleeping.

Lots of us have learned to "sleep on it" before making a decision. Recent scientific research has demonstrated that this old saying has a sound basis in fact. Researchers showed that people were able to improve their performance of a learned task after sleep. The researchers were also able to demonstrate that it was one particular type of sleep, REM sleep, which caused the improvement, because if sleepers were prevented from getting that particular stage of sleep, their performance did not get any better. So sleep naturally helps to improve our memory and performance, and with a bit of positive direction we can make it help us even more. Below, I will show you how to do that.

I just have to explain one thing first. It is important to put any request that you make to the unconscious in positive terms.

Let me show you what I mean. Try not to think of a blue elephant. Now, notice you can't help thinking of one before you put it out of your mind.

This is why it isn't useful to think about what you don't want, and why you should rather focus on what you DO want.

Of course, we live in a strange culture that is fascinated with problems and forgets to focus on the positives. So very often when I ask people what they want, I get a list of everything they want to move away from, like "I don't want to be fat" or "I want to stop biting my nails." The first thing I have to do is to get them to think in positive terms, like "I want to be slim" or "I want to be healthy" or "I want to grow beautiful, long nails."

So when there are things you are trying to achieve, and you don't yet know how you will achieve them, use this exercise.

Asking the Unconscious Mind to Help You

Read this exercise through carefully before you do it.

1. Before you go to bed, sit quietly for a few moments and think about the goal with which you want some help.

2. Formulate a request for your own unconscious that is simple. Don't ask for lots of things at once. If necessary, break down a big goal and deal with one bit at a time. Make it one short sentence.

3. Make sure your request is positive, for example, not "I don't want to fail my exam" but "I want to remember all I have learned."

4. Make sure your request is clear—have a clear picture in your mind of what you will be able to do when you get it.

5. When you have a simple, positive, clear request, repeat it a few times to yourself with your internal voice, then go on and go to bed.

For more practice in asking your unconscious for help, play the video "Getting Your Unconscious Mind to Help You Sleep."

This exercise will also help you to sleep better by addressing more of the hopes or concerns that used to keep you awake. Using the last two exercises makes sure there is no need to stay awake and worry—in fact, it sets you up so that your problems are even being sorted out while you sleep.

In a Nutshell

SORT OUT YOUR WORRIES DURING THE
DAY—SET SPECIAL TIME ASIDE TO
ORGANIZE YOUR THOUGHTS.

KEEP PEN AND PAPER BY THE BED TO
MAKE A NOTE OF GREAT IDEAS THAT
COME TO YOU AS YOU RELAX.

IF YOU ARE BOTHERED BY FEELINGS,
MAKE SURE YOU RECEIVE THEIR MESSAGES.

• • •

CHAPTER 8

•

What to Do If You Are Still Awake

What to Do if You Are Still Awake

I am giving you a selection of four different techniques here. Try them all out to find out which one works best for you. You won't need to do all of them every night, but you have to try each one to find out which is best for you.

As your sleep improves, you will find that it happens more and more easily and more and more automatically, but it is really useful to have these techniques if you need some extra help to let go of an unusual or stressful day. So practice each of them until you know them by heart and can use them without referring to the book.

All of these exercises will help you fall asleep more easily. The more you use all of them, the more you will find that you fall asleep quicker and more easily, and more and more often you'll be asleep before you get around to using them. Some people quickly find a favorite, others find they prefer using different ones on different nights. And some people like using a sequence of two different exercises.

Releasing the Day

For many people, going to bed is actually the first time since they got up when they can really relax, and sometimes you haven't had the opportunity to register all the events of the day and let it all soak in. That can cause you to go over and over things in your mind.

The very best way to deal with this problem is simply to go over all the events in reverse order so that each and every event is acknowledged and your mind can process all the emotions. This is how to do it.

Release the Day

Read this exercise through carefully before you do it.

1. In your mind, visualize what you were doing just before you went to bed.

2. Visualize what you were doing just before that—who was with you, what was happening.

3. Go back through the day, one event at a time, in full color and remembering all you heard and said.

4. For each event you will have a memory that is compressed—it won't take as long to remember it as it took to do it. But there will be a sequence, and all the key emotions will come back to you.

5. Go back through each event until you end up where you woke up this morning.

6. Now you know what happened, what you felt, and what you expected, and your mind can put them all together.

For a more in-depth exercise, play the Releasing the Day video.

Thought Field Therapy

Thought field therapy (often shortened to TFT) was created by my friend Roger Callahan. It looks a little unusual, but many scientific studies show that it's amazingly effective at reducing stress, trauma, and compulsion. Dr. Callahan discovered that specific patterns of tapping on key acupuncture points of the body have a rapid, reliable, and predictable effect on our feelings. His discovery brings together a modern scientific approach and the ancient understanding of the originators of acupuncture. Simply by using a series of taps in specific places on the body we can reduce the intensity of an emotion or feeling of stress and establish calm relaxation.

When people are stressed it's difficult to sleep. Sometimes people are stressed about the very thought of not being able to sleep, which makes them more stressed so they stay more awake. It's a vicious circle.

This technique is not merely a distraction. Scientific studies have shown that when we use the tapping technique we reduce stress chemicals in our body and produce states of relaxation. We also change the way our brain processes stress information. This makes it easier to sleep. The effect of tapping in the specific sequence I will share with you is to reset the way your brain interprets and responds to stress, altering your internal brain structure.

There is a particular pattern of tapping that reduces stress and anxiety, which is perfectly suited to helping you sleep when you are stressed about being awake.

Tapping into Your Natural Ability to Sleep

Read this exercise through carefully before you do it. After you have practiced this tapping sequence several times you will know it by heart.

Before you start, just notice how much stress or anxiety you feel. I'd like you to rate your stress about not being able to sleep on a scale of 1 to 10, with 1 being the lowest and 10 the highest. This is important, because in a moment we will want to know how much you've reduced it.

Now take two fingers of either hand and tap about ten times on each of the following points on your body while you continue to think about being unable to sleep:

Tap above your eyebrow.

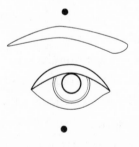

Tap under your eye.

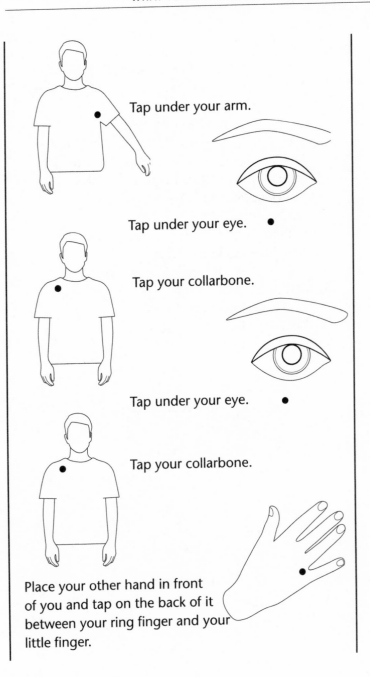

Tap under your arm.

Tap under your eye.

Tap your collarbone.

Tap under your eye.

Tap your collarbone.

Place your other hand in front of you and tap on the back of it between your ring finger and your little finger.

Continue to think about what it was like not being able to sleep as you do this and each of the steps that follow:

Close your eyes and open them.

Keep your head still, keep tapping your hand, and look down to the right then down to the left.

Keep tapping and rotate your eyes 360 degrees clockwise, and now 360 degrees counterclockwise.

Remember to keep thinking about the stress of being awake as you do this.

Now hum the first few lines of "Happy Birthday" out loud.

Count out loud from 1 to 5.

Once again hum the first few lines of "Happy Birthday" out loud.

Tap above your eyebrow.

Tap under your eye.

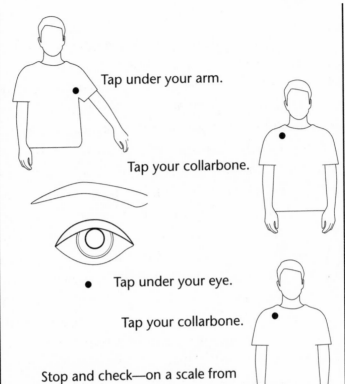

Tap under your arm.

Tap your collarbone.

Tap under your eye.

Tap your collarbone.

Stop and check—on a scale from 1 to 10, how do you rate your stress now at the thought of being awake?

If there's hardly any there, congratulations. If it has not reduced enough yet, just repeat the tapping sequence until it does.

If you feel now that the anxiety or stress is minimal or has completely gone, you may find you are too sleepy to concentrate on any more exercises. If you are tired but not yet completely sleepy, listen to the hypnotic trance or do one of the other exercises below.

To be guided through a tapping sequence, play the video "Tapping into Deep Sleep."

Internal Imagery

I came across this next technique quite by chance. Dr. Win Wenger is a researcher who specializes in increasing human intelligence. He explained to me a technique he uses to help people boost their IQs. Our minds are constantly processing a stream of images, sounds, and feelings. He discovered that when we describe out loud this stream of images it increases our intelligence by creating more complex neural networks in our brains. However, something very interesting happened when his research team described their image stream to themselves silently with their internal dialogue. When they were not speaking out loud, they found it impossible to stay awake. Some of the researchers could only stay awake for a few minutes, others managed a little longer, but over and over again they found themselves falling asleep in spite of their best efforts to stay awake.

As soon as I read about this, I knew I had to try this experiment with some insomniacs. It was amazing—some of them found that they fell asleep within a couple of minutes, others found it took a little longer or a little practice, but every single one found it transformed their experience of going to bed. They simply knew they were going to sleep, and they did.

Like anything, the more you practice it the better you get. So if you find yourself awake and you want to go to sleep, all you have to do is the following exercise until you can't stay awake any more.

Do NOT do this next exercise if you are driving or operating machinery. Only do it when and where you can safely relax completely.

Stop Your Mind from Racing

Read this exercise through carefully before you do it. Memorize it so you can do it in bed without having to refer to the book.

- Close your eyes and use your internal voice to describe to yourself silently whatever you are aware of. Give your internal voice a slow, relaxing monotone. For example:

  Now I see the ocean.

  Now I hear the crashing of the waves on the beach below me.

  Now I see the setting sun glinting on the waves far out to sea.

  Now I am aware that I hear the sound of my friend's voice.

  Now I am aware I see a swimming pool.

  Now I can see a giraffe.

  Now I see a bowl of oranges, and I remember the taste of orange juice.

  Now I can hear the sound of a car.

  Now I can feel the sun on my body . . .

  and so on.

- No matter how bizarre the things are that come into your mind, just carry on describing them in a continuous stream with a monotone voice. Remember the tone of your voice has a powerful effect upon your feelings. Allow your internal voice to gently murmur a description of almost everything that comes into your mind, just drone on and on, and you'll find your mind drifting and very soon wanting to nod off.

- If you are still awake a few minutes after starting this process, then you need to do two things. First, make your voice even more monotonous as you describe your experience, and secondly, keep doing it and doing it and doing it. If you do this properly it is absolutely impossible to stay awake.

For more practice, play the video "Stop Your Mind Racing and Become Calm."

Nighttime Waking

Some people find they get to sleep comfortably, but they wake up during the night and find it difficult to get back to sleep. There are several reasons why this happens. Eating too late and drinking too much alcohol can cause people to waken. Other causes are stress or pain or worry or sleep apnea. We addressed all of these problems earlier and have seen how to deal with them.

However, with some people I found that even when we dealt with these problems they were still waking up in the night. Sometimes the cause was simply that the sleep cycle was set too high, so instead of going back to sleep after a phase of REM sleep, they woke up.

Other times it seems that your unconscious is considering something while you are in REM sleep and it wants to show it to the conscious mind. When you've seen it, you can go back to sleep.

I realized that what was needed was an exercise that did two things. First, it had to let the unconscious show you something if necessary, and secondly it needed to mimic the process of REM to restart the basic sleep pattern. The important point is to give the conscious mind the role of observer instead of controller, and to free the unconscious mind to express itself however it wants. That is what this next exercise does. It gives your unconscious mind an opportunity to communicate with you through symbolism. As you become aware of the symbols, tension is released. You don't need to understand them, just let them be processed by both parts of your mind. The free association of this exercise parallels the REM process which tells your unconscious mind it is appropriate to go to sleep.

You can do this exercise when you go to bed, but it is particularly useful when you have awoken in the middle of the night.

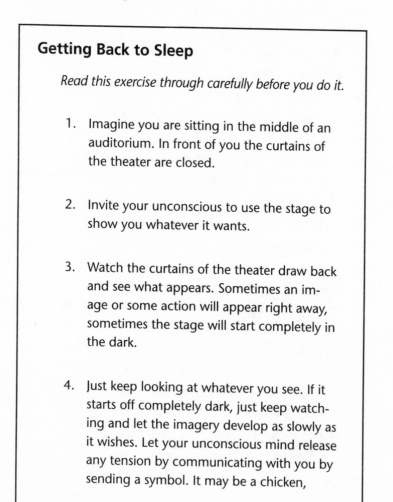

Getting Back to Sleep

Read this exercise through carefully before you do it.

1. Imagine you are sitting in the middle of an auditorium. In front of you the curtains of the theater are closed.

2. Invite your unconscious to use the stage to show you whatever it wants.

3. Watch the curtains of the theater draw back and see what appears. Sometimes an image or some action will appear right away, sometimes the stage will start completely in the dark.

4. Just keep looking at whatever you see. If it starts off completely dark, just keep watching and let the imagery develop as slowly as it wishes. Let your unconscious mind release any tension by communicating with you by sending a symbol. It may be a chicken,

a missile, an orange. It doesn't matter. Just
acknowledge the symbol and let the lights
fade.

5. Keep watching. Let another image arise.
    There is no need to understand or interpret
    what you see. Equally, if you do get some
    meaning from it, that is fine too. Just let
    your unconscious show you as much as it
    wishes.

6. If you feel that your mind is especially ac-
    tive, you can now combine this with "Stop
    Your Mind from Racing," describing what
    you are seeing with your internal voice in a
    gentle monotone, or you can simply carry
    on watching as you drift into sleep.

To see more of what your unconscious wants to
show you, play the video "Getting Back to Sleep."

Sometimes people tell me something they have re-
membered from this exercise and neither of us has any
idea what it means. Sometimes we find out later, and
sometimes we don't. It seems that, just like dreams,
sometimes the imagery is meaningful and sometimes
it isn't. But even when dreams do look meaningful,
remember that they are not factual statements. They
are imagery that can always be interpreted in several

different ways. The positive advantage of this exercise is not what you see, but simply the process of letting the images arise, letting yourself notice them, and letting them pass. As you get more and more used to it, the path into sleep becomes more and more straightforward.

• • •

CHAPTER 9

•

Summing Up

Summing Up

Q. HOW CAN I STOP RELIVING BAD THINGS THAT HAVE HAPPENED DURING THE DAY?

Of course we can't control everything that ever happens to us, but we do have a considerable amount of control over how we think and feel. When you do the psychological exercises in the book, like "Reducing Your Worries" (page 77) and "Letting the Feeling Unfold" (page 104), you will change your feelings about what took place today. You cannot go back and change the past, but you can absolutely change how you are feeling about things right now. If you feel you need to be calmer still, use the "Tapping" technique (page 118), which works wonders for any leftover stress of the day.

Q. I'VE GOT A BIG EVENT COMING UP AND MY MIND KEEPS GOING OVER IT, AND I KNOW I WON'T BE ABLE TO SLEEP TILL IT'S OVER—HOW CAN THIS SYSTEM HELP ME?

Your mind wants the event to go well, so the intention of running over it again and again is to make it as good as possible. However, sometimes our minds tend to overdo the job. That's all that is happening. However, something amazing occurs when we make a list of everything we can do to make something go well. Making the list acts as an acknowledgment and instruction to the unconscious mind. When you have listed everything you can do and made a note of when you will do it, use the "Reducing Your Worries" exercise (page 77). If there is any residual stress after that, use the "Tapping" technique (page 118).

Q. MY SHIFT SCHEDULE AT WORK CHANGES, SO IT'S IMPOSSIBLE TO HAVE A SET GOING-TO-BED OR WAKING-UP TIME—WILL THE SYSTEM STILL WORK IF I CAN'T REGULATE MY SLEEPING TIMES?

Every shift schedule is a schedule—even if only for a week. So apply exactly the same rules and make sure you listen to the hypnotic trance on the first night of every new shift schedule. Also, if you need to sleep during the daytime, make sure your bedroom is really dark and quiet, or use an eye mask and earplugs.

Q. I'VE ALWAYS BEEN A LIGHT SLEEPER. THE SLIGHTEST NOISE WAKES ME. CAN THIS SYSTEM HELP?

Just because you have been a light sleeper doesn't mean you have to be one in the future. This sounds like something you've believed about yourself and have reinforced. If you follow all the instructions in this book and regularly use the hypnotic trance, it's almost certain that you will sleep more deeply. Listen to the hypnotic trance every night when you go to bed, and if you wake during the night use the "Getting Back to Sleep" exercise (page 126). Soon you will be able to think of yourself as a much better sleeper.

Q. I GET WOKEN SEVERAL TIMES DURING THE NIGHT BY MY CHILDREN—HOW CAN I RELAX ENOUGH TO GET TO SLEEP AGAIN QUICKLY AFTERWARDS IF I'M REGULARLY DISTURBED?

When you go back to bed use "Systematic Relaxation" (page 88) and then "Stop Your Mind from Racing" (page 123). If you feel agitated, use the "Tapping" technique (page 118).

Q. IF THE KIDS HAVE KEPT ME UP AT NIGHT, I NAP DURING THE DAY BUT FEEL CONSTANTLY EXHAUSTED. IS NAPPING ALLOWED? I FEEL THIS IS MY ONLY CHANCE OF GRABBING SOME SLEEP.

If you are tired enough to sleep at night as long as you can, then nap during the day. Unfortunately the book can't stop the kids from waking you up at night!

Q. I FIND I CAN ONLY SLEEP AFTER I'VE HAD SOME ALCOHOL—CAN THIS SYSTEM HELP ME SLEEP WITHOUT IT?

Definitely! Remember alcohol may put you to sleep but it also can wake you up later. You will be amazed that even by the second night without alcohol you will actually sleep better. There is nothing wrong with drinking in moderation, but if you feel you need to have it to go to sleep, that is a problem, because the alcohol is in charge and not you. As you go the first few nights without a drink, it will feel different, but the hypnotic trance and the "Tapping" technique (page 118) are excellent for helping the body to readjust its chemistry. If you were using alcohol to get to sleep, that is like using crutches to walk. When you throw away the crutches, your legs take a few days to regain their full strength. Remember, only go to bed when you feel sleepy, and if you are unsure about your ability to go to sleep, use the "Tapping" technique (page 118) and "Systematic Relaxation" (page 88) when you go to bed and listen to the hypnotic trance. If you are worried about waking during the night, remember you can use the "Getting Back to Sleep" exercise (page 126).

Q. I'VE BEEN TAKING SLEEPING PILLS FOR SOME TIME AND AM WORRIED THAT IF I STOP TAKING THEM AND START USING THIS TECHNIQUE, I'LL GO BACK TO LYING AWAKE FOR HOURS.

You should only stop taking medication in consultation with your doctor. Your doctor will give you a program to help you reduce your medication very, very gradually. If you follow this program while you are reducing your medication, it will soon help you to sleep far better than before.

Nevertheless, if you have been using sleep medication for years, you may experience some sleep disruption while your body chemistry is readjusting. That is one reason why doctors insist that any reduction in medication is done very slowly. Remember you must always consult your doctor if you want to make any change to your prescribed medication.

Q. MY UPSTAIRS NEIGHBORS KEEP ME AWAKE NIGHT AFTER NIGHT, WHILE MY PARTNER SLEEPS THROUGH THE RACKET—HOW IS THIS POSSIBLE? CAN THIS SYSTEM HELP ME LEARN TO IGNORE IT?

Your partner knows that your neighbors are a nuisance but are not important—that is why he or she can sleep through the noise. You are probably angry with your neighbors, so it is not just the noise that's keeping you awake. The more you think about them the more you will notice it. Even as you get into bed, you are probably already listening for noise from your neighbors and are commenting to yourself about them and winding yourself up. You can ask your neighbors to be quieter, but even if you can't change them, you can change how you feel. Use the "Tapping" technique (page 118) to reduce the anger, and then listen to the hypnotic trance when you go to bed so you have something welcome to listen to.

Q. I'M CONSTANTLY WORRIED ABOUT PEOPLE BREAKING IN. HOW CAN I RELAX ENOUGH TO GET TO SLEEP?

This is a good example of your mind overprotecting you. We should all be concerned about security, so it is useful to ask yourself, "Is the house safe? Did I forget to lock the front door? Did I turn off the gas?" However, if your mind is repeating those worries over and over again, you just need to lower the thermostat of concern.

First of all, do check the front door is locked and so on, then use the "Reducing Your Worries" technique (page 77). Then listen to the hypnotic trance.

Q. WHY DO I WAKE UP SO EARLY?

You may be one of the people who naturally need only five or six hours' sleep. It doesn't matter if you wake early so long as you are truly refreshed.

Q. I'M EXHAUSTED WHEN I COME HOME FROM THE OFFICE, BUT COME BEDTIME, I'M WIDE AWAKE—WHAT CAN I DO?

Your mind is tired from working, but your body has not had enough exercise. Remember, exercise is very efficient at washing the stress toxins out of your body, and if you do it three or four hours before you go to sleep, it helps you to sleep deeper. So when you get home, do some exercise. It could be something as simple as a brisk walk for 20 minutes. This will help to match your mental exhaustion with some physical tiredness. Remember, also, to follow the rules and don't go to bed until you are sleepy. For one or two nights it will be quite late before you are really sleepy and can then go to bed, but your system will soon readjust to the correct cycle, and after a few days you will find you are sleepy at the right time.

Q. THE ONLY WAY I CAN GET TO SLEEP IS IF I LEAVE THE TV ON, BUT IT THEN WAKES ME UP IN THE EARLY HOURS—WILL THIS SYSTEM HELP?

Remember, you should never watch TV in bed. Also remember that you should turn the TV off an hour before you go to bed. And finally, don't go to bed until you feel sleepy. It may be that the first one or two nights you end up going to bed much later than you expected, but within a few days you will be sleeping better, deeper, and longer than before.

Use the hypnotic trance when you get into bed and you will reprogram your mind to fall asleep quite naturally. You can also use "Stop Your Mind from Racing" (page 123) to assist the process.

Q. I'M WORRIED THAT IF THIS SYSTEM WORKS TOO WELL, I WON'T HEAR MY CHILDREN IN THE NIGHT IF THEY NEED ME. WILL I STILL WAKE UP IF I'VE BEEN LISTENING TO THE HYPNOTIC TRANCE?

Yes, every mother knows that she can be in the deepest sleep and if her newborn baby makes the slightest noise she is awake.

Even though you are asleep there is still a part of your mind that's always listening. The sleeping patterns we are restoring are your natural way of sleeping, so you will always be able to respond to your natural instinct to care for your child and to wake up when necessary.

Q. SOMETIMES, JUST AS I'M DROPPING OFF, I GET PANIC ATTACKS, AND NOW I FEEL I'M TOO SCARED TO LET MYSELF RELAX COMPLETELY.

Panic attacks are simply emotional messages that are being delivered too loud and too fast. Your emotions are trying to help but are happening so fast that you cannot receive the message they are delivering. As soon as you get the original message, the panic attacks will no longer be necessary. Use the "Letting the Feeling Unfold" technique (page 104) to find out what the message is. When you have discovered the simple positive intention of the feeling, your body will be able to relax. If at first it feels a bit strange being truly relaxed, use "Systematic Relaxation" (page 88) to start yourself off.

You can also use the hypnotic trance that contains suggestions to help you relax and to ensure that you can wake when necessary.

Q. MY RESTLESS LEGS KEEP TWITCHING AS I'M DROPPING OFF, WHICH KEEPS ME AWAKE—CAN THIS SYSTEM HELP?

There are several causes of restless leg syndrome. For some people it is a symptom of the release of the stress from the day. All the elements of this sleep system will help to reduce the symptoms. It is also particularly helpful to ensure you get some exercise during the day. If you still feel some symptoms, you can let it happen several times before it stops, or you can shake the leg yourself in the same motion. When you make the motion deliberately yourself you begin to take control of the muscle memory, and then you can begin to reduce the shaking little by little until the leg is completely relaxed. If you "take over" like this each time it happens, gradually you will reset the muscle memory to bring your legs to relaxation.

If you have any concerns about your symptoms, you should always consult your doctor.

Q. WHY DO I WAKE UP IN THE
MIDDLE OF THE NIGHT?

Your natural sleep cycle is being disrupted so that when your brain waves come up into REM sleep you waken before you return to deep sleep. This can happen for many reasons, including drinking too much alcohol or too much water or having undischarged stress or trying to go to sleep too soon. Make sure you have made a note of all the things on your mind before you go to bed and use the "Reducing Your Worries" technique (page 77), and remember, only go to bed when you are sleepy. If you find yourself awake in the middle of the night, use the exercises "Systematic Relaxation" (page 88) and then "Getting Back to Sleep" (page 126).

Q. WHY AM I HAVING TROUBLE
MAKING THIS WORK?

You are not following all the instructions. Although natural healthy sleep is actually very easy, people accumulate all sorts of bad habits by accident that can interfere with the sleep cycle. It is difficult to tell in advance what are the particular causes of any one person's insomnia. Therefore you must follow every single one of the rules and use all the exercises and the hypnotic trance and your sleep will improve. You may be one of the people who only need five hours' sleep, but when you follow all the instructions, those five hours will be deep and refreshing and you will wake with all the energy you need for the whole day.

• • •

The Golden Rules of Sleep

All you need to set yourself up for a wonderful night's sleep every night.

1. Get up regularly half an hour earlier than your usual desired getting-up time.

2. Go to bed only when you are sleepy.

3. Don't take any naps during the day.

4. At least three times a week, get at least 20 minutes of exercise.

5. Finish eating at least three hours before you go to bed.

6. Don't have any caffeine after 2 P.M.

7. Cut out alcohol.

8. Switch off the TV one hour before you go to bed.

9. Do only three things in bed: sleep, make love, and use this book or the hypnotic trance.

10. If you are awake in bed for more than 20 minutes, do one of the exercises (see the index opposite) or get up and do something boring.

11. Keep your bedroom dark at night.

12. Have a warm, comfortable bed in a room that is not too hot.

13. Don't watch the clock.

14. Use the hypnotic trance.

• • •

INDEX OF TECHNIQUES AND EXERCISES

1. *Reducing Your Worries* — 77
2. *Practicing Being Drowsy* — 79
3. *Calming the Internal Voice* — 85
4. *Systematic Relaxation* — 88
5. *Changing Your Story* — 92
6. *Value Yourself* — 96
7. *Letting the Feeling Unfold* — 104
8. *Asking the Unconscious Mind to Help You* — 109
9. *Release the Day* — 115
10. *Tapping into Your Natural Ability to Sleep* — 118
11. *Stop Your Mind from Racing* — 123
12. *Getting Back to Sleep* — 126

• • •

A FINAL NOTE

So that's the system. Now that you have read this book, you have all you need to change your sleeping patterns for the better.

However, you will definitely find it helpful to read this book several times so that you don't miss anything, and to practice the techniques until they become second nature. Remember also to use the hypnotic trance regularly whenever you need to reinforce your sleep cycle.

Often people tell me that they read one of my books to change a particular area of their life and they found several other areas of their life improved significantly as well.

A human being is an interdependent system, and as your sleep improves you are more rested, more energetic, and more creative, so it is reasonable to expect that your whole life benefits. May you live the life you want and exceed your expectations!

Good night and God bless.

Until we meet,

Paul McKenna

• • •

ACKNOWLEDGMENTS

Dr. Richard Bandler, Dr. Roger Callahan, Kate Davey, Dr. Natheera Indrasenan, Robert Kirby, Michael Neill, Dr. Hugh Rienhoff, Mari Roberts, Dr. Ron Ruden, Dr. John Sotos, Clare Staples, Dr. Win Wenger, Doug Young, and all the clients with sleep problems I have worked with over the years who have taught me so much.

Finally to Dr. Hugh Willbourn, a personal and professional inspiration, but more than that, a good friend.

• • •

We hope you enjoyed this Hay House book. If you'd like to receive our online catalog featuring additional information on Hay House books and products, or if you'd like to find out more about the Hay Foundation, please contact:

Hay House, Inc., P.O. Box 5100, Carlsbad, CA 92018-5100
(760) 431-7695 or (800) 654-5126
(760) 431-6948 (fax) or (800) 650-5115 (fax)
www.hayhouse.com® • www.hayfoundation.org

• • •

Published and distributed in Australia by:
Hay House Australia Pty. Ltd., 18/36 Ralph St., Alexandria NSW 2015
Phone: 612-9669-4299 • *Fax:* 612-9669-4144 • www.hayhouse.com.au

Published and distributed in the United Kingdom by:
Hay House UK, Ltd., Astley House, 33 Notting Hill Gate, London W11 3JQ
Phone: 44-20-3675-2450 • *Fax:* 44-20-3675-2451 • www.hayhouse.co.uk

Published and distributed in the Republic of South Africa by:
Hay House SA (Pty), Ltd., P.O. Box 990, Witkoppen 2068
info@hayhouse.co.za • www.hayhouse.co.za

Published in India by: Hay House Publishers India,
Muskaan Complex, Plot No. 3, B-2, Vasant Kunj, New Delhi 110 070
Phone: 91-11-4176-1620 • *Fax:* 91-11-4176-1630 • www.hayhouse.co.in

Distributed in Canada by: Raincoast Books,
2440 Viking Way, Richmond, B.C. V6V 1N2
Phone: 1-800-663-5714 • *Fax:* 1-800-565-3770 • www.raincoast.com

• • •

Take Your Soul on a Vacation

Visit www.HealYourLife.com® to regroup,
recharge, and reconnect with your own magnificence.
Featuring blogs, mind-body-spirit news, and
life-changing wisdom from Louise Hay and friends.

Visit www.HealYourLife.com today!

Free e-newsletters
from Hay House, the Ultimate
Resource for Inspiration

Be the first to know about Hay House's dollar deals, free downloads, special offers, affirmation cards, giveaways, contests, and more!

 Get exclusive excerpts from our latest releases and videos from **Hay House Present Moments**.

 Enjoy uplifting personal stories, how-to articles, and healing advice, along with videos and empowering quotes, within **Heal Your Life**.

 Have an inspirational story to tell and a passion for writing? Sharpen your writing skills with insider tips from **Your Writing Life**.

Sign Up Now!

Get inspired, educate yourself, get a complimentary gift, and share the wisdom!

http://www.hayhouse.com/newsletters.php

Visit www.hayhouse.com to sign up today!

     HAYHOUSE RADIO *radio for your soul®*   HealYourLife.com ♥

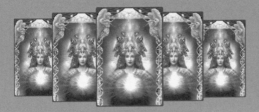

Paul McKenna, Ph.D., is described by Ryan Seacrest as "a cross between the Dr. Phil and Tony Robbins of Britain." Recently named by the *London Times* as one of the world's leading and most important modern gurus, alongside Nelson Mandela and the Dalai Lama, he is Britain's best-selling nonfiction author, selling 8,000 books a week in 35 countries—a total of 8 million books in the last decade. He has worked his unique brand of personal transformation with Hollywood movie stars, Olympic gold medalists, rock stars, leading business achievers, and royalty. Over the past 20 years, Paul McKenna has helped millions of people successfully quit smoking, lose weight, overcome insomnia, eliminate stress, and increase self-confidence. Dr. McKenna has appeared on *The Dr. Oz Show, Good Morning America, The Ellen DeGeneres Show, Rachael Ray, Anderson Live,* and *The Early Show.* He is regularly watched on TV by hundreds of millions of people in 42 countries around the world.

Dr. McKenna has consistently astounded his audiences and clients by proving how small changes in people's lives can yield huge results, whether it's curing someone of a lifelong phobia or clearing up deep-seated issues in a matter of minutes. He currently hosts his own TV show on Hulu, where he interviews the most interesting people in the world. His guests include Simon Cowell, Harvey Weinstein, Rachael Ray, Sir Roger Moore, Roger Daltrey, Tony Robbins, Paul Oakenfold, and Sir Ken Robinson. Website: www.mckenna.com

**FOR MORE INFORMATION
GO TO
mckenna.com**

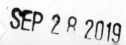